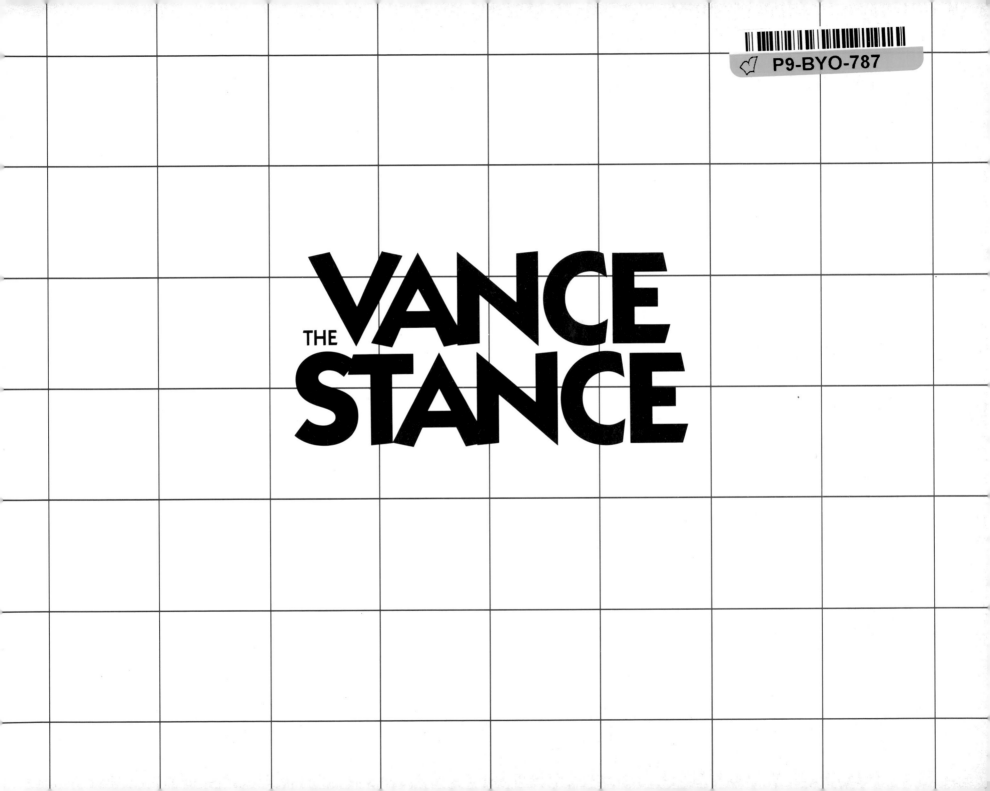

THE VANCE STANCE

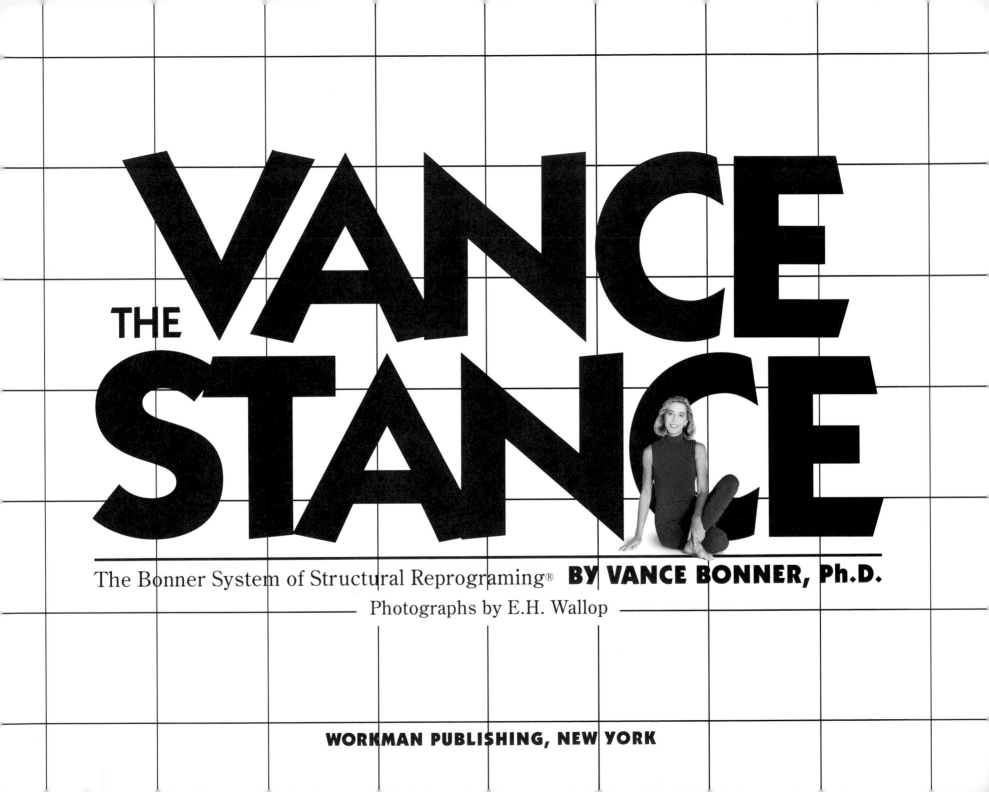

The Bonner System of Structural Reprograming® **BY VANCE BONNER, Ph.D.**

Photographs by E.H. Wallop

WORKMAN PUBLISHING, NEW YORK

Library of Congress Cataloging-in-Publication Data

Bonner, Vance.
The Vance Stance / Vance Bonner.
p.   cm.
ISBN 1-56305-311-X (PAP) : $10.95
1. Stretching exercises. 2. Posture. 3. Health. I. Title.
RA781.63.B66   1993
613.7'1—dc20   92-50281 CIP

Workman books are available at special discounts when purchased in bulk for premiums and sales promotions as well as for fund-raising or educational use. Special editions or book excerpts can also be created to specification. For details, contact the Special Sales Director at the address below.

Workman Publishing
708 Broadway
New York, NY 10003

Printed in the United States
10 9 8 7 6 5 4 3 2 1

This book is lovingly dedicated to my wonderful mother, who always told me I was capable of accomplishing anything I wanted to; and to the memory of my dear father, who had lovely posture and who suggested that I might have the same.

It is also dedicated to all of my clients and friends who believed in me enough to let me work with their wonderful bodies, who trusted me long enough to get the point, and who were generous enough to let me share in the joy of their transformations. Their continued requests for a book prompted me to undertake this project.

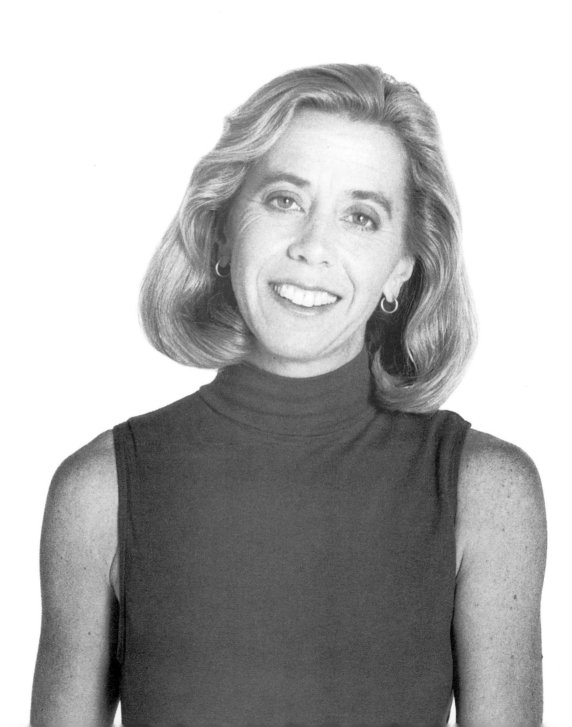

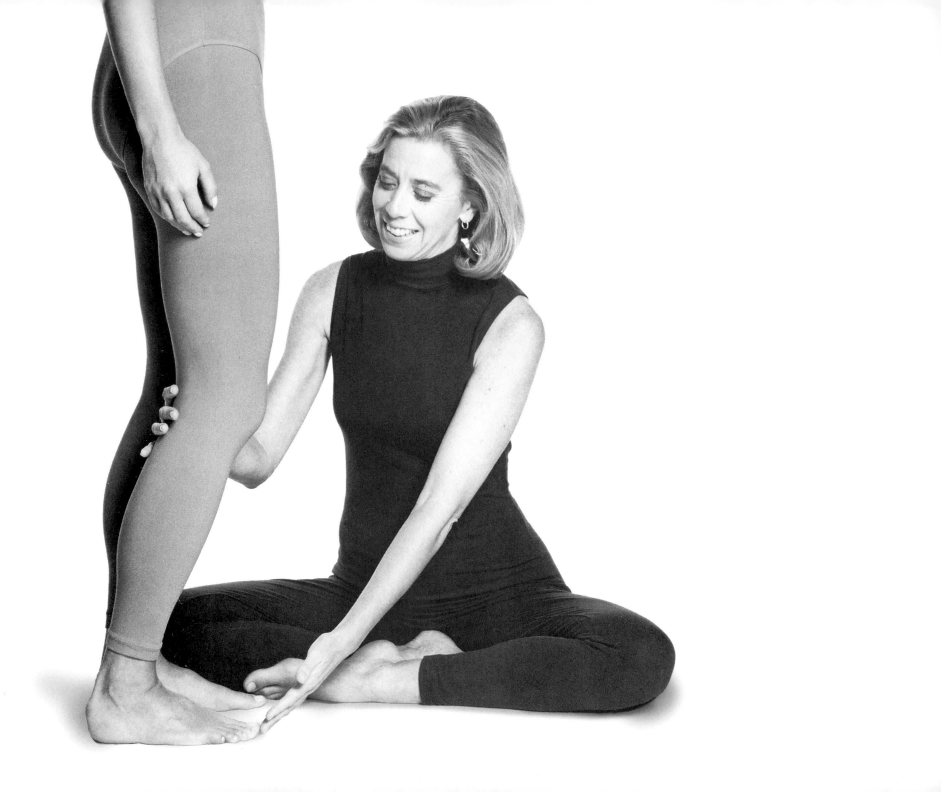

There are many people to be thanked for helping to make this book a reality.

First and foremost, my eternal thanks to my sister-in-law, Beth Bonner, for lovingly transcribing the entire original manuscript to computer disk, editing word-by-word as she went. She transformed the hunt-and-peck-typed rough pages into a cohesive whole. Her enormous support at the early stages made the daunting task possible.

Thanks to Peter Workman and Sally Kovalchick for their courage and foresight in presenting a work that does not fit an existing niche and for persevering until we got what we all wanted. Thanks to everyone at Workman for participating so fully in the Stance, wherever we did it, and particularly to Carolan Workman for her enthusiasm and kind words always. Thanks also to Lisa Eskow for her great assistance in the early going, Carbery O'Brien, and to Steve Jenkins and Stuart Henley for the fine appearance of the book.

Special thanks to Carol Saltus for her grand work on the text.

I am grateful to Drea Besch, Michael Castegnola, Mary Olsen Kelly, Emily Katz, Milian France, Candace Wheeler, Sherrie Connelly, Julianne Blake, Pamela Shandel, Karen Rubin and Peg Pearson for doing the movements as they were read aloud; to Leona and Jerry Schecter, who believed in the work and made valiant attempts on my behalf; to Janice Gherke and Pat Setter, who pioneered the Canadian workshops; and to the many original clients who assisted me in the early days, including Jeannie Waller and Gloria Garfunkle in New York, Ellie Reed, Shari Hunt Brown and Bill Innes in Sun Valley, Julie Firestone in Phoenix, and Joyce Taylor and Hal and Sidra Stone in Los Angeles.

Many thanks to Scott Riklin for helping finalize the deal (and for great therapy over the phone!); to Tommy Hutton for the original tapes; to Larry Becker for dragging me to that important meeting; to Pam Ritsau and Pam Tunno for brochure input; to Nita Alvarez for the best brochure; to Ruth Avergon for her love and constant support; to the founders and members of The Inside Edge, my "extended family of choice"; and to Master Bong Soo Han, the Black Belts and students at Hapkido, for many years of personal challenge and growth.

Thanks especially to The Shadow, my canine constant companion, for teaching me unconditional love and the pleasure of stretching. To the Religious of the Sacred Heart for exemplifying so well the true meaning of *educare* and for teaching me how to think and look at things from a new perspective, I offer my love and heartfelt thanks.

Above all, thanks to my family for years of encouragement and help, especially to Carolyn Bates Bonner for editing along the way and to Mark Healy Bonner, Esq., for all his assistance in completing this work. Also to Gregory, Katharine, Christopher, Elizabeth, Jeanette, Ian and Emmett Bonner. I am proud to be related to you.

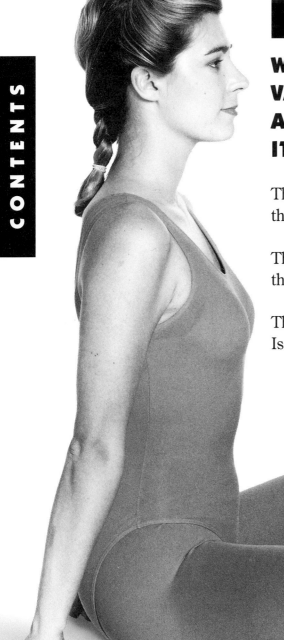

CONTENTS

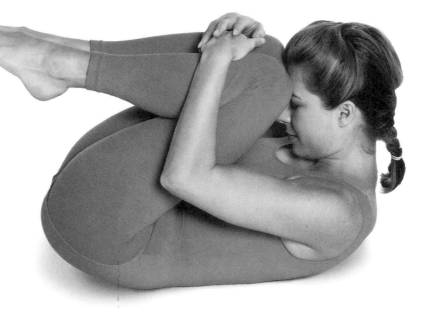

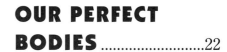

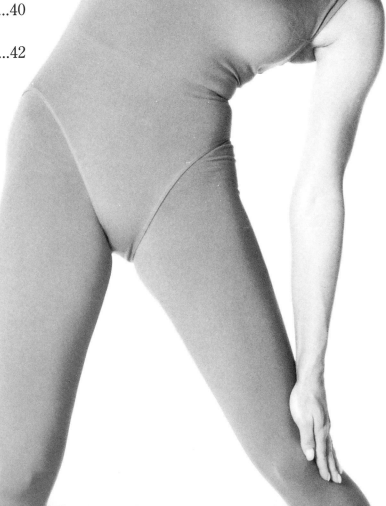

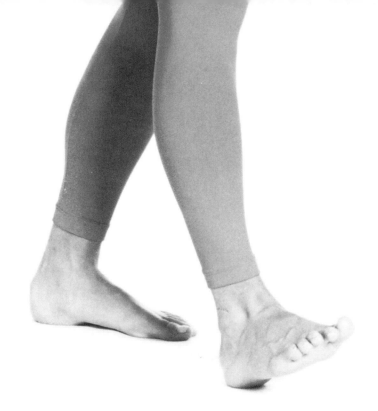

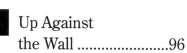
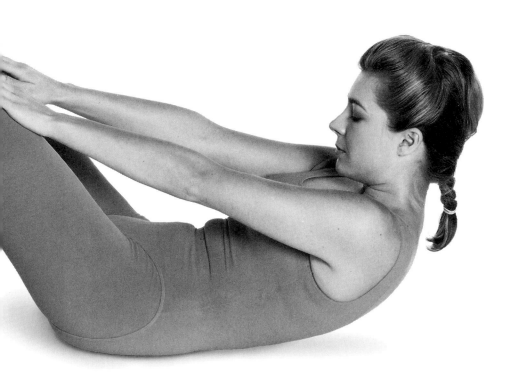

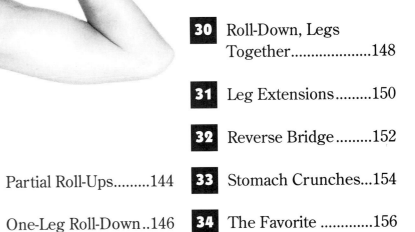

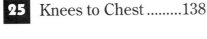

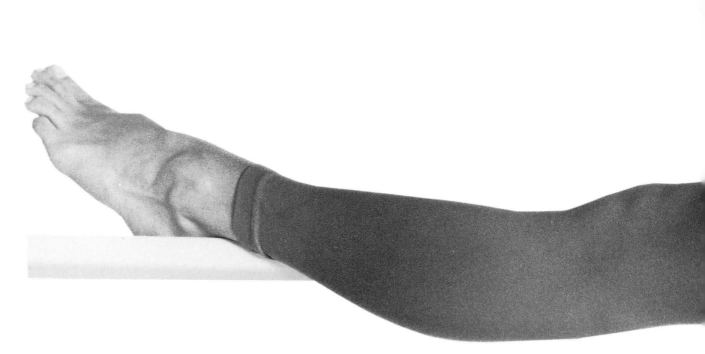

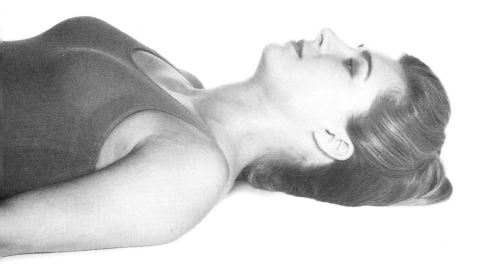

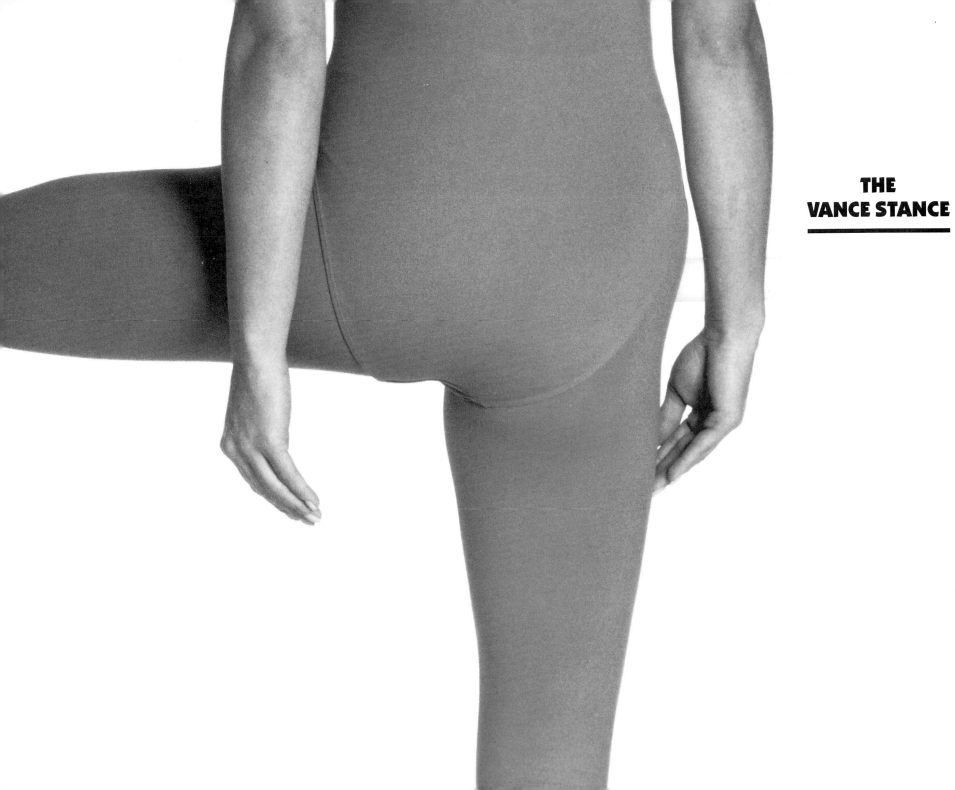

WHAT IS THE VANCE STANCE— AND WHAT CAN IT DO FOR YOU?

When I began teaching flexibility classes twenty years ago, I found that my students tended to be so tight in the hamstrings (the muscles that run up the backs of the legs) that they couldn't touch the floor with their legs straight; some could barely bend over. I noticed, too, that almost all of them habitually stood with their knees locked back, rather than lightly flexed, loose and easy, ready to move.

These same students also had swaybacks, and they all complained of lower back pain. As soon as we released and stretched those tight muscles in their legs, the pain in their lower back started to ease. I realized then that the tightness followed a pattern: the people who were the most contracted in the legs were the tightest in the small of the back.

But why, I wondered, did this particular pattern of tightness in the legs cause pain in the lower back? Then I understood. It was the way they were holding their *spine*—the whole length of the spine—in relation to their *feet* that determined the degree of tension in the lower back. That is, the more out of alignment

they were, the more likely they were to have lower back pain. It seemed logical that if the spine

Proper alignment gives your body the maximum possible range, strength and ease.

and legs were repositioned, or realigned, relative to each other, then pressure on the lower back would be relieved—and so would the pain.

I therefore began to work on changing the alignment of the body as a way of alleviating *back pain*. Furthermore—and this was crucial—it was the alignment of the *entire body* that was involved, beginning with the soles of the feet and extending all the way up through the legs, the torso and the head.

I soon saw the benefits of this work dramatically demonstrated in my classes. People with chronic back pain that had been steadily worsening for years were now able to resume activities they'd almost forgotten they were ever able to engage in.

People who had seemed almost deformed, so twisted were their bodies, began to stand tall and straight. People who had had repeated orthopedic surgery and been told to give up hope of ever again playing tennis, or skiing, or even driving a car, were back on the court, the ski slopes and the road. And people who seemed irrevocably condemned to a continuing, even accelerating skid downhill through the "aging process"— who were stooped, shuffling, dim shadows of what they'd once been—became rejuvenated as though by magic.

THE PRINCIPLES OF THE VANCE STANCE

For the first time, my students were standing and moving in the *correct relationship to gravity*. They were able to ease the grip of muscles that were never meant to be held so tense and contracted, so that their bodies, now released, could maintain themselves easily, lightly and freely upright.

When we lock our knees, a habit we learn in childhood, we immediately pull our center of gravity back, out of the correct placement. This forces us to tighten in the lower back, thrusting it forward and shortening and deepening its curve, in order to counterbalance the locked-back knees. And this backward and forward thrust alternates all the way up the body. We curve back in the upper spine in order to counterbalance the forward thrust of the lower back (the swayback), and then the shoulders pull forward, and the head correspondingly pulls back. We form a series of "S" curves—short, tight, compressed—all the way up from feet to head. Certainly, all this effort and distortion just to keep our balance, to keep from pitching forward on our faces, could not be what Mother Nature had in mind for us.

THE NATURAL WAY

Observing this virtually universal pattern among my students, a pattern that caused so much restriction, tension and pain, started me on a quest to learn how our bodies were meant to be used. I wanted to know why so many of us cannot stand and move without discomfort and fatigue, why we tend to lose our bodily strength and flexibility so inexorably and steadily as we grow older, whether or not these losses are avoidable—and what Mother Nature really had in mind for us when she 'designed us as she did.

What I discovered led me to develop the Vance Stance, a program that will show you 1) a very different way to use your body right now, 2) that it is indeed the *way* you use your body that is causing you pain and trouble, 3) how to recognize and change old habits of use for new ones that work for you instead of against you, and 4) how to maintain and enhance this new way of using your body in everything you do.

I have found that, without a doubt, how we move and hold ourselves is largely responsible for most of the pain that we experience. Old, unconscious habits of misalignment, never detected and thus never corrected, directly cause muscle and joint pain, fatigue and general bodily difficulty. Most of us don't realize this crucial connection, much less know what to do about it. The Vance Stance will let you experience the fact that there *is* another way to stand and move. With awareness, you will learn how to choose this better way.

BALANCE IS THE KEY

The Vance Stance teaches *Balanced Alignment,* a way of positioning the body in space that will enable you to stand and move with both grace and power. First you'll learn what you've been doing wrong, then you'll "reprogram" yourself for new, balanced and therefore effortless and easy ways of standing and moving. You'll learn to recognize and correct old habits of misuse that cause chronic pain, limitation, and loss of flexibility and strength that are usually associated with aging—but that often begin as early as age twenty-five or thirty.

The Vance Stance substitutes balance for stress and effort in the way you use your body in every aspect of your life. You work *with* instead of *against* gravity, so that your body maintains itself effortlessly in space. When each section of your body is properly placed relative to the rest, you don't have to strive to hold yourself up against the downward pull of gravity; the sensation is rather of being sustained on an upward-flowing *stream of energy*.

With the simple techniques of the Stance, you will learn how to achieve Balanced Alignment and

The Stance enables you to work *with* gravity instead of against it.

17

maintain it in everything you do. All your patterns of movement will be more elegant and efficient as you eliminate both the causes of bodily stress and its harmful effects. You'll move more lightly and gracefully than ever before, with many new possibilities open to you in every activity, at work and at play, as your power and endurance increase.

THE PROMISE OF THE VANCE STANCE

Together we will evaluate your present postural habits, and I will show you how to correct them according to the principle of Balanced Alignment. You will then learn the series of Thirty-Four Movements that will enable you to integrate this new way of holding yourself in space, of "being-in-your-body," into every aspect of your life.

After practicing the Stance and the movements, even for a short time, you're likely to notice that you're in better shape now than you were even ten years ago. You'll have more energy and a deeply satisfying sense of hope that you can actually change and even *improve* with age. Chronic problems such as sciatica and "runner's knee" will vanish as

their causes are eliminated. You'll know how to stand and move without fatigue. You'll have a new control of your body, with a new awareness that will enable you to correct as well as prevent bad habits that cause pain and limitation. You'll be inspired to become more active, to take up new sports or resume those you once enjoyed. And you'll be preparing your body to "age" with undiminished resilience and vigor.

I can promise you that many of your fears of aging will vanish, too. In fact, you'll probably redefine for yourself what aging means; you'll realize that so many of the problems of aging have nothing to do with years lived, but rather were caused by unconscious habits of posture and movement that are completely correctable. You'll face the years to come with new anticipation and hopefulness.

The increase in life expectancy that we've been promised by the end of the century—to well over a hundred years!—is more a threat than a promise unless our level of well-being is radically improved at the same time. If we're already feeling pain at forty or fifty, what will it be like to be

still on our feet at ninety or a hundred? Who *wants* to live to a hundred and twenty if our last forty or fifty years are spent with a walker or in a wheelchair?

What we look forward to is not prolonged years of debility, but the pleasure in living some of our best years, extended by decades. The Vance Stance can make that possible by showing how to substitute power-enhancing postural habits for the damaging ones that can only lead to progressive deterioration.

THE VANCE STANCE IS FOR EVERYONE

Because its principles are universal and serve us from the beginning of life to its end, the Vance Stance benefits everyone, from children to centenarians. My oldest client is one hundred and three! The next senior are ninety-six and eighty-nine; many are in their eighties, seventies and sixties. Many, too, are professional athletes in their twenties and thirties.

New postural habits will change the look of your body.

How can the same principles benefit both a professional ice skater whose triple axels have begun to falter and a waitress whose main complaint is having to stay on her feet all day? A tennis player with tendonitis and a salesman who spends hours in the driver's seat? Because Balanced Alignment, the principle behind the Stance, underlies *everything we do,* whoever we are. This single, unifying anatomical law is basic to the way all of us function best, whether we're washing dishes or turning cartwheels. And the simple exercises included in the Vance Stance program are not calisthenics but a means of preparing the body to apply this principle to daily living.

The Vance Stance provides a total system of control and harmony in movement. If you choose the way of perfect balanced alignment, through the techniques of the Vance Stance, you can establish a relationship between your body and gravity that is one of lightness and ease.

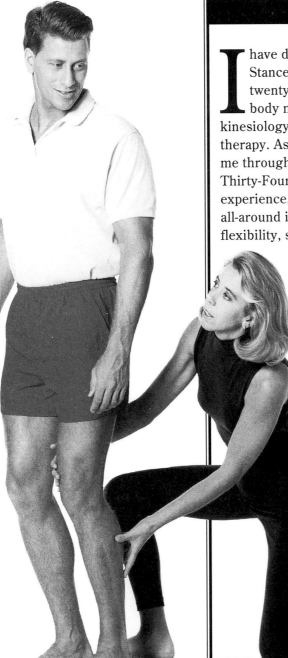

Balanced Alignment begins with correct placement of the feet, ankles and knees.

THE VANCE ADVANTAGE

I have developed the Vance Stance over more than twenty years of teaching body mechanics, kinesiology and exercise therapy. As you progress with me through the Stance and the Thirty-Four Movements, you'll experience, step by step, the all-around improvement in flexibility, strength, confidence and hope that this program promises. The Vance Stance:

- Replaces harmful, constricting, stressful postural habits with liberating correct ones.
- Locates and then eliminates the causes of chronic joint and muscle pain.
- Restores your awareness of underused muscles and develops overall muscular elasticity and strength, offering you greatly increased skill and pleasure in everything you do.
- Increases strength, improves flexibility, and enhances balance and grace in persons of all ages. Your body will have an energy and a resilience you may never have known before.

Once you've mastered the two parts of the Vance Stance—the Stance and the movements—you will look and feel better (the very shape of your body may undergo a radical improvement!) and you will possess a new strength and flexibility.

The Vance Stance is unique. It differs from other exercise programs in that:

- It provides a grid, an objective tool, for measuring and assessing exactly where you are in relation to the ideal of Balanced Alignment and what you need to do to achieve it.
- Using the discoveries about yourself and what you must do in order to correct harmful postural habits, it offers you the program of Thirty-Four Movements that strengthen weak muscles and releases those that are tight so that it becomes easy and natural to live in Balanced Alignment.
- Unlike other programs, limited to all-purpose calisthenics that are not custom tailored to meet your specific needs, it identifies your individual problems and suggests specific exercises aimed at correcting them.
- It can benefit everyone, no matter the age or level of conditioning.

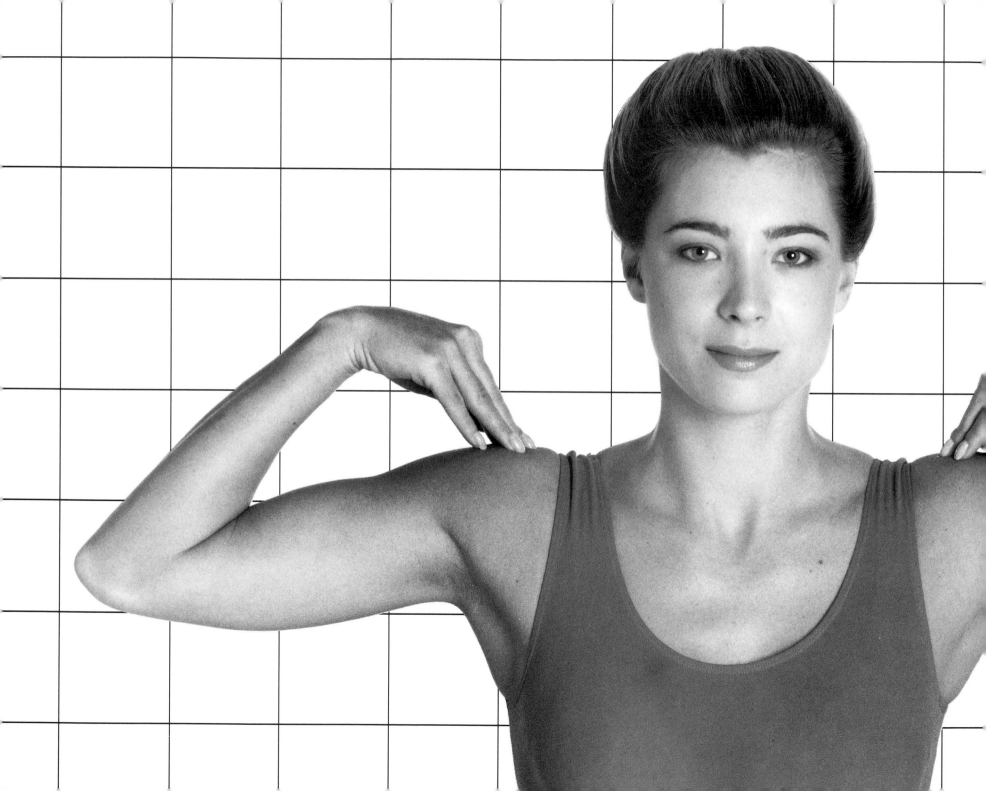

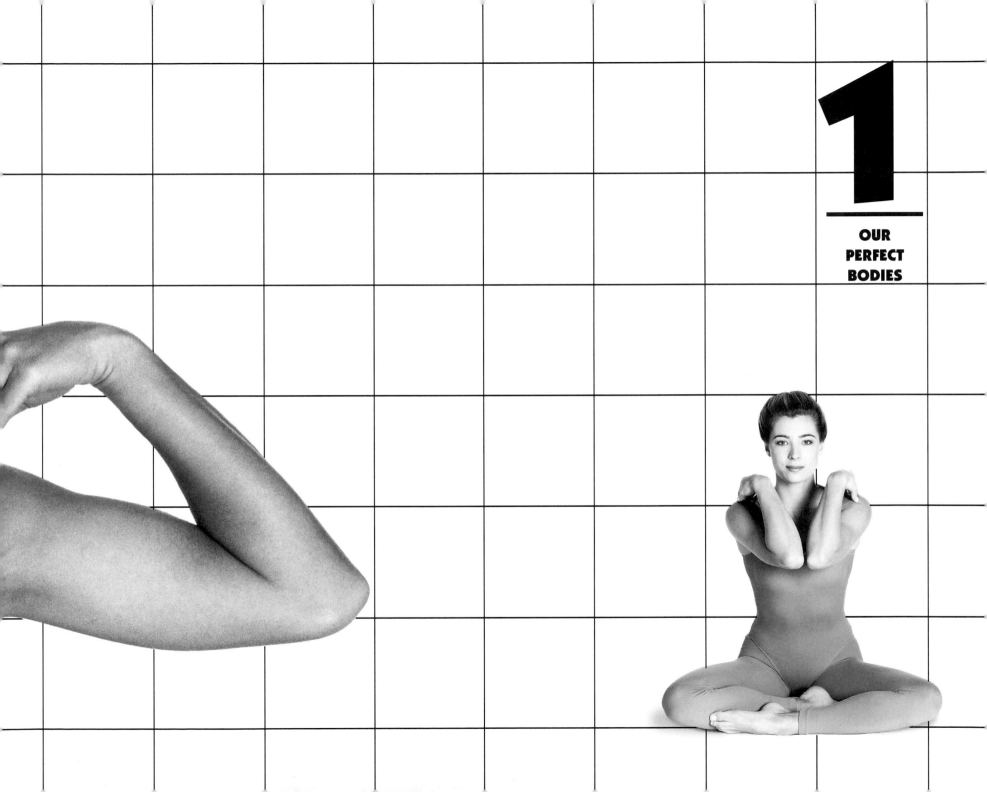

1

OUR PERFECT BODIES

Most of us take our bodies for granted. We expect them always to do what we ask of them, effortlessly and efficiently; we assume that they will always be there for us. And so we go through our daily lives thinking about anything and everything except how we use these reliable vehicles, these loyal servants that unquestioningly carry out all our orders.

Until, that is, something goes wrong—a knee "goes out," or a hip, a shoulder or back. We experience tension and fatigue in making the simplest movements. We suffer chronic or acute, even crippling pain. Why? Oh, just bad luck, we say, or heredity ("Weak knees run in my family"), or an old injury "acting up." Or, that catch-all explanation, the "aging process." After all, isn't it a known fact that aging means loss—loss of strength, of endurance, of resilience?

Somewhere behind this pessimistic view lurks the notion that we have to pay for having gotten up from all fours, back at the dawn of evolution, and that most of our ailments—pain, fatigue, stiffness, weakness— are an inevitable cost of erect posture. But the truth is, these ailments are not inevitable or even normal. We *can* advance into maturity with unimpaired and even enhanced flexibility and strength—as we were meant to. We were endowed at birth with bodies that are perfectly designed to serve us with ease and enjoyment through a long, active and pain-free lifetime.

So what goes wrong?

What we think of as the inescapable toll of some vague "aging process" has in fact two very specific causes. The first is *misalignment*, or an unbalanced relationship of the parts of the body—and of the body in relation to gravity. The second is *loss of flexibility*, or loss of freedom and mobility—of the full range of motion of the muscles and joints. In other words, we sit, stand and move crookedly, and we do it more and more stiffly and tightly. And, owing to a third factor, *loss of awareness*, we don't even realize we're doing these things, which makes it impossible to correct them.

We marvel at other perfectly functioning machines, such as a beautifully tooled car, but we tend to overlook the most wonderful machine of all— the human body. Blessed with phenomenal powers of regeneration, our bodies can withstand years, even decades, of systematic misuse and still continue to serve us faithfully, with only the occasional twinge or ache, or a knee or back that "goes out" periodically. And then, when the years of punishment have finally taken their toll, we resign ourselves to "getting old." Our bodies are "old," and we no longer expect pain-free service from them— or that they will be as strong and resilient as they were when we were younger.

But this is simply adding insult to injury. Age is not the problem. It's the piling up of years of abuse—of driving the car with the brake on and without changing the oil, so to speak. And to an amazing extent, once we become aware of what we're doing to ourselves and begin to use our bodies the way they were designed to be used, the damage of all those years can be halted, and healed.

OUR IDEAL SELVES

No, our upright posture does *not* mean that as we grow older we must expect fatigue, stiffness and pain. On the contrary, by getting up from all fours, we've gained the capacity for a freedom, a versatility, denied to other animals. But our upright posture, with all its advantages, does carry with it a certain responsibility. The parts of the body must be aligned in space, maintaining their relationship not through effort but through balance. And we are in a state of perfect skeletal and muscular balance when gravity exerts no uneven downward pressure on any part of us. I call this relationship Balanced Alignment.

This optimum state of Balanced Alignment depends on *maximum length*. "Length, length, and more length" is the slogan in my classes. When we stand as tall and as straight as possible, not bent or tilted or twisted, when the resting length of our muscles is as long as possible and our joints as free as possible, we are in Balanced Alignment.

Length, in turn, depends on *flexibility*. And flexibility is what we're likely to lose fastest as we grow older—or after a period of inactivity—unless we maintain and enhance it by regularly stretching our muscles and keeping our joints open and free in their full range of motion.

BALANCED ALIGNMENT

When, somewhere back in our beginnings, we decided to rise up on our hind legs and balance on two feet, we surrendered the automatic balance enjoyed by an animal that stands supported squarely on four feet, as steady as a table. Such an animal is in a state known as "stable equilibrium," which can be disturbed or shifted only by a powerful force.

We are extended far into space, straight up and on a very small base. But our feet, along with ankles that articulate, are the specific tools that allowed this posture. Longer than hooves or paws, they work with the ankles and back in an interplay so ingeniously engineered that we can choose among many different ways to move our bodies—options that are not open to other animals. True, we are fundamentally insecure, at least as far as standing on our feet is concerned. But this doesn't mean we have to live precariously, in constant danger of pitching forward on our faces. Rather, it requires a relationship with gravity founded on an easy balance, or equilibrium, in which no part of the body is fixed or locked and we are always free to

move, ready to respond quickly to any demand. In lightness and freedom, the parts of the body stacked up tall, riding easily on top of each other and each centered on the one below— this is how we should be aligned in space.

Correct alignment is never stiff or static; it is *dynamic,* allowing the greatest range of response, and it enables our bodies to work with gravity rather than having to struggle against it.

THE FRIENDLY FORCE OF GRAVITY

Gravity has gotten a bad name; we blame it for all our troubles in later life, as though we could live better without it. But we would not be ourselves without gravity. Our skeletal system developed in intimate association with the force of gravity. It is through the need to "stand up" to it, to overcome its pressure, that our bones develop their strength; without its pull, we immediately start losing bone mass. Just ask the astronauts of the earlier generation what it means to live outside the field of gravity. They often spent months weightless in space before it was realized what the consequences would

be, and all of them suffered severe bone loss. No one knew at the time that exercises must be devised for use in space in order to simulate the effect of the force of gravity on the body.

GO WITH THE FLOW

The force of gravity can be used to open the stopped-up passageways of the body. Like a drain opener that bubbles through a clogged-up drain in the sink, the downward pressure of gravity tends to add tension to any area in the lower half of the body that is tight or restricted.

Part of the reason such areas become tight in the first place is that proper pressure on them to remain open is withdrawn as the body shifts out of its correct alignment, interrupting the natural flow of energy.

So we are creatures of gravity and entirely dependent on it for our well-being, even our survival. The more we lock at the joints, keep our muscles tense and contracted even when they're not working, and compress the spinal column, the shorter and tighter the natural curves of our body become and the farther we deviate from the place where gravity can't hurt us. And, because we're standing and moving "crookedly," the more crooked (and therefore overbalanced) we are and the more effort it takes simply to stay on our feet.

In Balanced Alignment, each segment of the body is balanced above the one below, so that the line of gravity runs right through the center of each segment and no part is skewed or protrudes off the center line. All this must happen from the *middle* of the foot, not just the heel. Only by using the feet in very precise relation to the ankles, legs, back and head can we position the spine forward enough to experience what seems to be a reversal of gravity's pressure. It is the long, straight, released alignment of all the body segments, achieved through the Stance, that gives us the optimum energy and lift from the power of the gravity stream. Only *here* is there an absence of pressure and pain in the body.

MUSCLE POWER

What throws us out of alignment is an imbalance in the tension of muscles that are working to support or move us. Muscles work in pairs. The flexors are the pulling muscles, such as the biceps, or "Popeye" muscle, in the upper arm. The biceps contracts when you pull something toward you—a chair, for instance. The opposing muscle in the back of the arm, the triceps, contracts when you want to push the chair away from you. These muscles are in a balanced relationship when they are equally strong, and when at rest each is *as long as possible*. Regular stretching of the muscles is what gives them their maximum resting length. Stretching is also essential for muscle "tone," meaning the resilience and elasticity of the muscles.

The health of muscles, as well as the balance of opposing pairs of muscles, depends about equally on their ability to contract (shorten) and stretch

The Vance Program of movements is designed to strengthen weak muscles and release tight ones so that muscle pairs can work in proper balance.

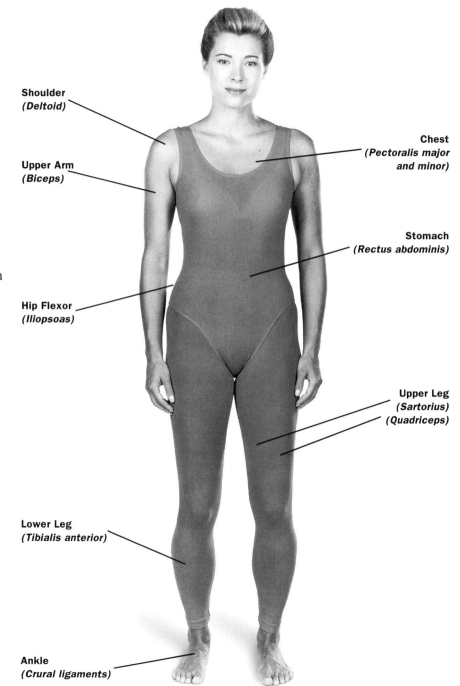

Shoulder
(Deltoid)

Chest
(Pectoralis major
and minor)

Upper Arm
(Biceps)

Stomach
(Rectus abdominis)

Hip Flexor
(Iliopsoas)

Upper Leg
(Sartorius)
(Quadriceps)

Lower Leg
(Tibialis anterior)

Ankle
(Crural ligaments)

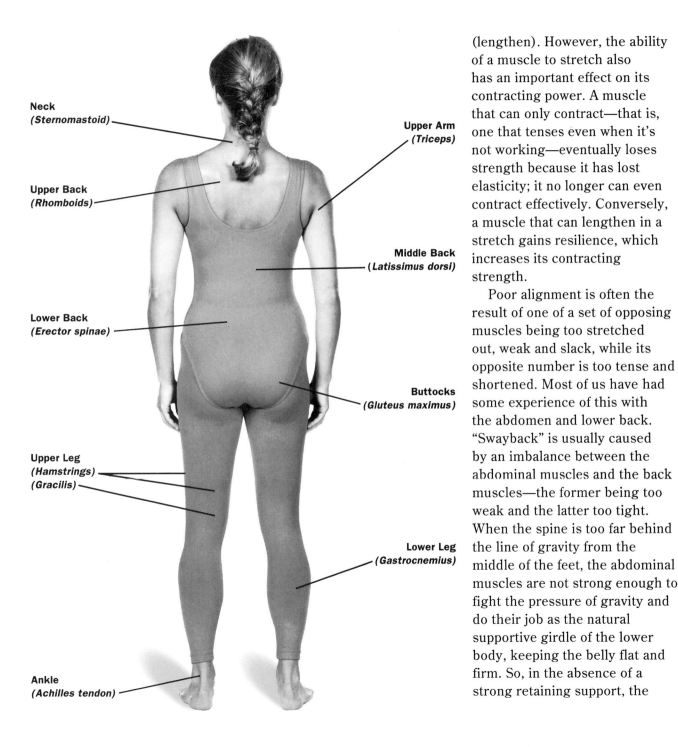

Neck
(*Sternomastoid*)

Upper Back
(*Rhomboids*)

Lower Back
(*Erector spinae*)

Upper Leg
(*Hamstrings*)
(*Gracilis*)

Ankle
(*Achilles tendon*)

Upper Arm
(*Triceps*)

Middle Back
(*Latissimus dorsi*)

Buttocks
(*Gluteus maximus*)

Lower Leg
(*Gastrocnemius*)

(lengthen). However, the ability of a muscle to stretch also has an important effect on its contracting power. A muscle that can only contract—that is, one that tenses even when it's not working—eventually loses strength because it has lost elasticity; it no longer can even contract effectively. Conversely, a muscle that can lengthen in a stretch gains resilience, which increases its contracting strength.

Poor alignment is often the result of one of a set of opposing muscles being too stretched out, weak and slack, while its opposite number is too tense and shortened. Most of us have had some experience of this with the abdomen and lower back. "Swayback" is usually caused by an imbalance between the abdominal muscles and the back muscles—the former being too weak and the latter too tight. When the spine is too far behind the line of gravity from the middle of the feet, the abdominal muscles are not strong enough to fight the pressure of gravity and do their job as the natural supportive girdle of the lower body, keeping the belly flat and firm. So, in the absence of a strong retaining support, the weight of the belly sags forward and pulls the lower back with it, shortening the muscles of the lumbar (lower) spine.

LENGTH, LENGTH, AND MORE LENGTH

Balanced Alignment is a natural state, not some artificial ideal. We begin life in perfect alignment; when we move out of gravity's lift and become misaligned, it is because the tension in the muscles that move our bones is uneven. This tends to throw us off balance, which leads to grabbing and locking in the joints, and to shortening and compressing the spine and all parts of the body in relation to the spine.

Here is the cause of most of our problems in using our bodies: when we are behind the lift of gravity, we need something to stabilize us, so we lock at the joints, tightening the muscles around them, and we compress the spine—basically in order not to fall. But this only pulls us farther off balance and stresses the joints, which results in our all-too-familiar back problems, bad knees, hunched or round shoulders and sagging stomachs.

The human body works best when the muscles are at their

longest possible resting length, with *the most distance between the joints* and *the greatest length in the spine.*

We achieve this length through the *balanced pull* of opposing muscles (as in the biceps/triceps example, or the abdominals and lower back) while in correct placement over the feet. Our work together will consist mainly in achieving this balanced pull: putting the body in this new place in gravity, and experiencing it long enough to find it again, by releasing and lengthening the overtight muscles and strengthening the slack, weak ones. Balancing the pull of muscles means that both sets of opposing muscles are as elastic as possible.

When this has been achieved, not only will you feel tall, straight and easily balanced, but you'll also experience an astonishing lightness, almost as though gravity has reversed itself and is lifting you up instead of pulling you down. You'll owe this exhilarating feeling to the fact that your muscles are no longer letting you down by being either too slack or too tight, wasting your energy, unbalancing you by pulling you back off the center of your feet; rather, they are

working together with maximum efficiency to support and carry you. Energy locked into overtight muscles is dammed up, blocked in the joints, and your body as a whole feels heavy, as if gravity were dragging you down. When muscles are balanced and free to stretch or to lengthen or shorten, the energy stream flows freely and gravity acts as a helpful, sustaining force.

Gravity is a *cooperative* force; it is not an enemy, bound to "get you" if you live long enough, but an indispensable friend. Gravity works best for us, however, when we're balanced *within its stream*, as straight and as long as possible, so that it cannot exert a downward pull on any single part of the body—as when we are out of alignment. In other words, gravity is a hostile force when we carry ourselves tight, locked or twisted, and a supportive friend when we are in Balanced Alignment.

FLEXIBILITY

Flexibility means freedom to shift forward at the ankles, to find the lift of gravity and to release the pull on our joints. We are freest when we are at our longest and straightest, but it's also worth emphasizing the

factor of flexibility in itself because it is so crucial in keeping us strong and pain-free. Far more than strength or endurance, which get called on only sporadically, our flexibility affects us from moment to moment in everything we do— yet it's what we lose first.

The body works most easily when used most correctly.

Flexibility of the joints depends on having muscles that are both strong and elastic, that can lengthen and contract to perform any movement we want. Our shoulder joints are free when our arms can swing freely forward, to the sides, back and down, in big, loose circles. Our hip joints are free when our legs can make the same large circles. The shoulder and hip joints both are ball-and-socket joints, which is why our arms and legs can make these circular movements. The knee, however, is a hinge joint, and so is the elbow; these can only extend and flex, open and close.

Freedom of movement is achieved through equalizing the tension of opposing sets of muscles. If one set is too tight while the other is too slack, the range of motion of the joint upon which these muscles act together to move it will be restricted. A good example is the upper back. "Round shoulders," which can look like a deformation of the bones, are actually caused by muscle imbalance. The muscles of the upper chest are too contracted and tight, while the upper back muscles are too weak, too stretched out. Instead of exerting a compensating pull, the upper back muscles yield to the stronger, tenser upper chest muscles, which pull the upper body forward without resistance. Because of the incorrect placement over the feet, and the resulting poor alignment, they have no alternative. And note that this tendency can only increase unless conscious effort is made to correct it; that is, the chest muscles tighten more and more as they continually act to pull forward, and the back muscles become more and more stretched as they are pulled forward. The way to correct this is to stretch the muscles of the upper chest, balancing their contracting power with lengthening, *and* to contract the muscles of the upper back, balancing their lengthening capacity with an equal contracting strength. We lengthen the short, tense muscles, and we tighten the long, slack muscles. Then the correctly aligned body is placed *with* gravity—to *stay* that way.

In the Thirty-Four Movements, we will do two kinds of work on muscles, *strengthening* them through movements that make them contract and *lengthening* them by stretching. Muscles are naturally elastic, like rubber bands, but we can greatly increase their elasticity by consciously doing stretching movements. This achieves the goal of *maximum resting length* for our muscles, so that when we are relaxed, our joints are completely open and free, and capable of their maximum range of motion. When our muscles are tight, our joints tend to be correspondingly stiff; the way to free and open the joints is to stretch the muscles that move them. You're as old as your joints—but it's in your power to keep them young!

"YOU'RE AS OLD AS YOUR JOINTS"

THREE MEN AND A MOUNTAIN

Perhaps the most astonishing—and rewarding—changes among my students can be seen in the older people. They have found out for themselves the truth of the idea that you *can* be getting better, not older.

One winter day I was standing atop Bald Mountain, admiring the view with three of my favorite senior students, aged seventy-two, eighty and eighty-five. We had come there to ski, and they were so alive and eager to have a good time that I was full of admiration for them.

We took off, playing follow the leader down the mountain until another group skied in front of us and forced us onto a trail used by kids who would dare each other to jump the bumps for the thrill of flying through the air and landing a long way off. I was in the lead, and as I hit one of these bumps and felt myself leaving the ground, I had a flash of terror. What would happen to my pals, who were following right behind me? Visions of broken legs, crutches and hip replacements raced through my head. But then, as we began landing one by one on the other side, the eighty-five-year-old shouted exultantly, "I haven't gotten this much air in forty years!"

At last I was convinced that it was literally true: there are no fixed limits, and even the most advanced years don't have to mean an end to adventure.

No one was hurt because we all knew how to take the impact of the jump and absorb it with our released and flexible joints. "You're as old as your joints," the saying goes, and these men all had joints that were far, far "younger" than their years. Their joints were both flexible and strong because they'd worked hard to get, and keep, them that way through their sessions with me.

They had all learned, in their bones, that dedicated stretching and the Balanced Alignment it allowed were the key to their body's youthful functioning. They were advanced in years but determined to continue advancing in the active lane; they would join no wheelchair and walker brigade. And here, in one dramatic moment, was their reward.

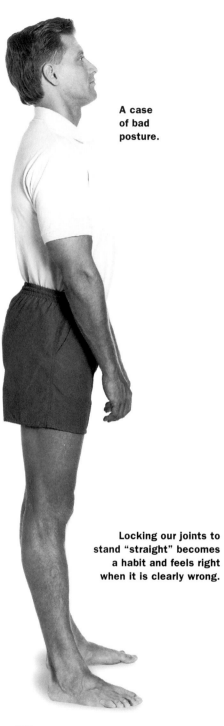

A case of bad posture.

Locking our joints to stand "straight" becomes a habit and feels right when it is clearly wrong.

28

IF WE WERE BORN PERFECT, WHAT HAPPENED?

As I walk down the street and look at the other pedestrians, I marvel at how distorted the human body can become. Seldom do I see a body that's perfectly aligned; when I do, it reminds me of what a marvelous machine we have at our disposal. Too often I see an imbalance in the body so radical that it's a wonder its owner is in motion at all. It appears that we can be pigeon-toed, knock-kneed, bowlegged, hunchbacked, have a shoulder or a whole side hiked up higher than the other, be bent over almost horizontal to the ground, or be twisted or tilted or both. Our backs—those extraordinarily flexible columns of nerve, bone, muscle and ligament—can be skewed out of line in so many directions, it's as though some malign imagination were at work thinking up ways to make them go awry.

MISALIGNMENT

If we were born with symmetry and balance, how does it happen that so often, by the time we're out of our thirties, our bodies feel like a burden we've been saddled with? Why do so many of us drag ourselves about so joylessly? Just "normal" wear and tear? No. The principal cause that I have observed in my work stems from the fact that we are all standing like two-year-olds.

The locked knee. Babies who first try to stand quickly discover that there is little strength in their legs to keep them upright. Instinctively, and ingeniously, the brain comes up with a quick approximation, a *compensation,* that involves deriving strength from locking the knee joints. This stabilizes the body, and the child is off and running.

doing it, this way of standing seemed to be perfectly acceptable and no one ever questioned its efficacy.

Now, however, we must step back and look at this instinctual response. Locked knees are the main source of misalignment and its attendant pain; we must learn a new way of standing that allows the body to work *within* the gravity stream.

Injury. A second cause of misalignment is injury to the body that results in a temporary "favoring" of one part over another. We tend to "protect" any part of the body that has been injured in order to shield it from

Locking your knees is the single most damaging thing you can do to your body.

The trouble is, locked knees provide an *artificial* means to an end—one that is only safe to use for a short time. Locking the knees places most of the weight back on the heels, forcing the entire body out of the flow of gravity. But since it worked for us as children, and we most likely saw our parents

further injury while it's healing. In time, the "favoring" may sink below the level of awareness, until the favored side becomes permanently weaker. We will see how this tendency to compensate for a temporary imbalance owing to injury becomes a problem when it has persisted past its usefulness as protection, when it has become unconscious habit that continues long after the injury has healed. (Incidentally, most injuries sustained in the course of normal activity result from misalignment. We tend to get hurt in a place that has been weakened because the muscles that support or move it are unbalanced.)

Habitual fixed position. Maintaining a habitual fixed position at work, or in the course of daily living, is still another cause of misalignment. Hunching over a computer, carrying a weight in one arm, wearing cameras slung over a shoulder, standing for long periods with the weight on one foot, sitting slouched—these positions tend to become stabilized by locking to relieve fatigue, which tends to "freeze" the locked joint or joints, which in turn become progressively immobilized. And the position becomes increasingly habitual, feels increasingly "natural."

Only with awareness of poor postural habits like those demonstrated here can we begin to reverse their damaging effects.

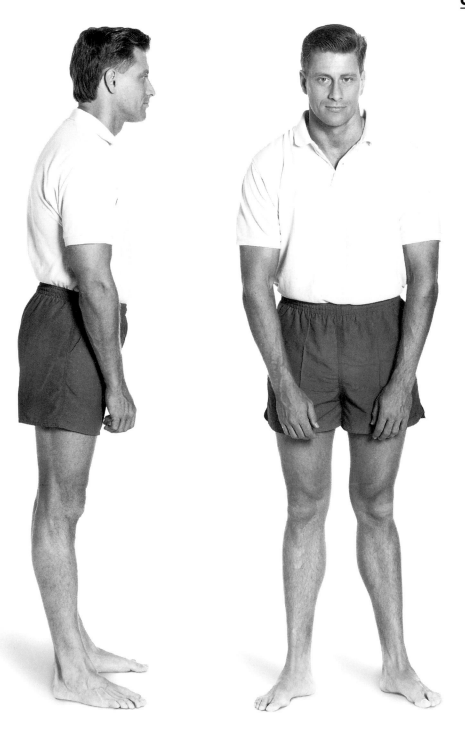

COMPENSATION

How is it, though, that these causes of misalignment (locked knees, injury and habitual fixed position) can get control of us—can feel so natural that after a time we're not even aware how far we've deviated from the ideal balanced alignment that is our natural endowment? Why does the wrong way stay with us and even come to feel more "right" than the true right way?

We owe this problem, in fact, to an extremely valuable innate ability—the body's ability to adjust to continuing stress. When, for any of the reasons given above, the body may be temporarily out of alignment, we still usually have to continue to use it. "Compensation" is the term for the body's ability to get the job done somehow, to keep us functioning even with one arm in a sling, ingeniously figuring out a way around this literally crippling obstacle. Our original compensation, locking the knees to give support to still-weak baby legs, set the stage for all the near-approximations to follow. The stress we felt from being pressed on by gravity was not supposed to last so long, and so we figured out a way to ignore the feelings of misalignment.

Suppose you have to keep your weight off an injured foot while it heals. You make the other foot take most of the weight that would normally be borne by both feet. Your body can adapt to this temporary loss of one of its two weight-bearing parts by making adjustments between its relationship to gravity and its own weight, so that one leg does most of the work of getting you around. But that's not all your body does for you in the way of compensation; it also makes this new way of walking as *comfortable* as possible—probably so you won't be tempted by discomfort to stress your injured foot and damage it further by making it bear weight too soon.

So your body does two things for you: it finds a way to keep you moving when part of your equipment is out of service, and in making this adjustment it sees to it that you experience minimum discomfort. Compensation can be described as an adaptive talent of the brain, which "figures out" how you can, in the above example, continue to walk when one foot is out of commission without feeling too much pain. The brain is able to switch you to an alternate mode of locomotion, automatically, when needed.

Let's take the more drastic case of a broken leg set in a heavy cast. Your body would instantly organize itself into unfamiliar patterns of weight-bearing to meet the demands of a new way of walking—and to yet another when the cast finally comes off and you're left with a temporarily atrophied, perhaps shriveled limb. The brain is able to take in two disparate pieces of information ("Right leg carrying fifteen-pound load, can't bend or take weight" and "Must get over to kitchen table") and, with no conscious thought on your part, to find a way of carrying out your needs under these new conditions.

Compensation becomes a problem only when you've become so comfortable with it—and furthermore, the injured leg, now healed, has become weak from disuse—that you keep limping or favoring the injured leg even when it's no longer necessary because this now feels like the "normal" way to walk. If you persist, one leg will eventually become shorter than the other, and soon limping will feel right and the normal way of walking would be uncomfortable, even painful. The same is true of hunching the shoulders or carrying one hip higher than the other.

Perhaps the most familiar form of compensation is the development of muscle strength to meet the demands of a heavy, uneven load. If you always carry a heavy bag in your right arm, for instance, the muscles of that arm and on that side of the chest (the obliques, which run from hip to armpit) will become stronger than the muscles on the left side. Unless you consciously balance the load, using the left

---

It's important to recognize habitual compensations that stand in the way of correct alignment.

---

side as often as the right, and also make a point of regularly stretching out the muscles on the right, you'll become permanently contracted toward that side; this means that even when you're carrying nothing, you're likely to be out of alignment, with your right side visibly shorter than your left.

Through this process of compensation, any of the causes of misalignment discussed earlier can bring about a situation where the misaligned state feels "natural," "right," "just the way I am," the body accepting it as the norm it has to work with. While extremely inefficient, this compensated state is at least bearable— for a time.

THE GRACE PERIOD

In any mechanical system, components that are positioned incorrectly cause excessive wear on other moving parts. An automobile engine whose piston timing is off will run, but only at the cost of strained internal parts, wasted fuel and, eventually, mechanical breakdown. Similarly, the body can continue to operate for a while with improperly aligned moving parts before the extra

friction begins to damage the system. During this "grace period," the time that elapses between adaptation to the incorrect alignment and the incorrect alignment and the

point at which actual damage occurs, the body compensates for—seemingly adjusts to— the strain caused by the misalignment. When you were a teenager, for example, you probably seemed almost to thrive on junk food and next to no sleep. In fact, you weren't thriving, but you could get away with it—your young body could handle almost any demand. But finally, after years and years of misuse, during which we exploit to the full the body's powers of compensation, the body notifies us that the grace period has expired by sending us signals

of pain. Pain is a warning that something is wrong and a request that we pay attention.

Many people respond to this warning signal by taking pain-

Pain is not the result of aging, or bad luck, or heredity. It is always a warning that something is wrong.

killers. These eliminate the pain, temporarily, but do nothing about its cause. If we think of pain as vital information, we'll think twice about getting rid of it before we try to trace this urgent message to its source. Most of my clients come to me because, gradually or suddenly, they have become unable to do things that once were easy— a young skater is no longer able to land his triple axels, a traveling salesman can't sit behind the wheel as long as he used to—and this rebellion of the body usually is signaled by acute or chronic pain.

The pain may be experienced only sporadically at first. Among my clients, I've found that after the first bout of pain, which usually comes sometime in the mid-twenties, the pain tends to recur more and more frequently and more insistently over the years. It's as though the body were saying, "Listen to me! I'm telling you that something is wrong! Pay attention and fix it!"

When the cause of the misalignment is not corrected— when we fail to change what we're doing with ourselves, usually because we no longer realize what it is that we're doing—we'll be sent more and more pain, more and more often, so that eventually attention will *have* to be paid. There are few attention-getters more effective than having your back "go out" on you, so that you have the choice of either lying rigid or being wracked with muscle spasms. Now, however, with the Vance Stance, you have a new choice. You can either block this urgent communication with painkillers, or you can listen to it and decide to change.

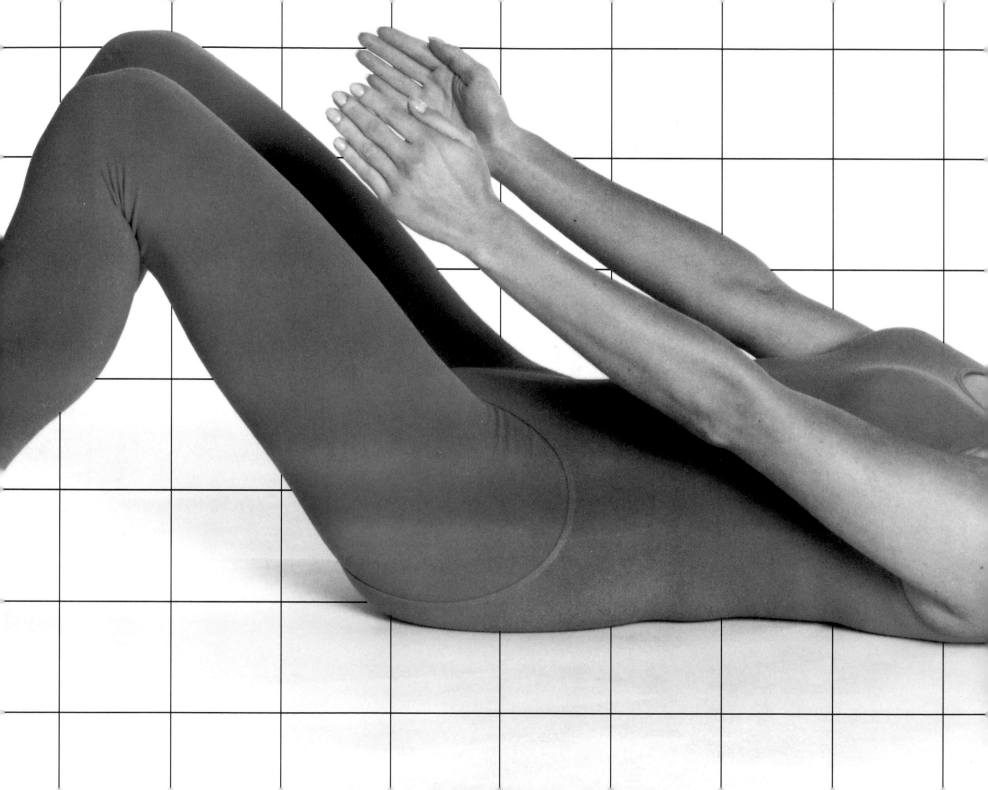

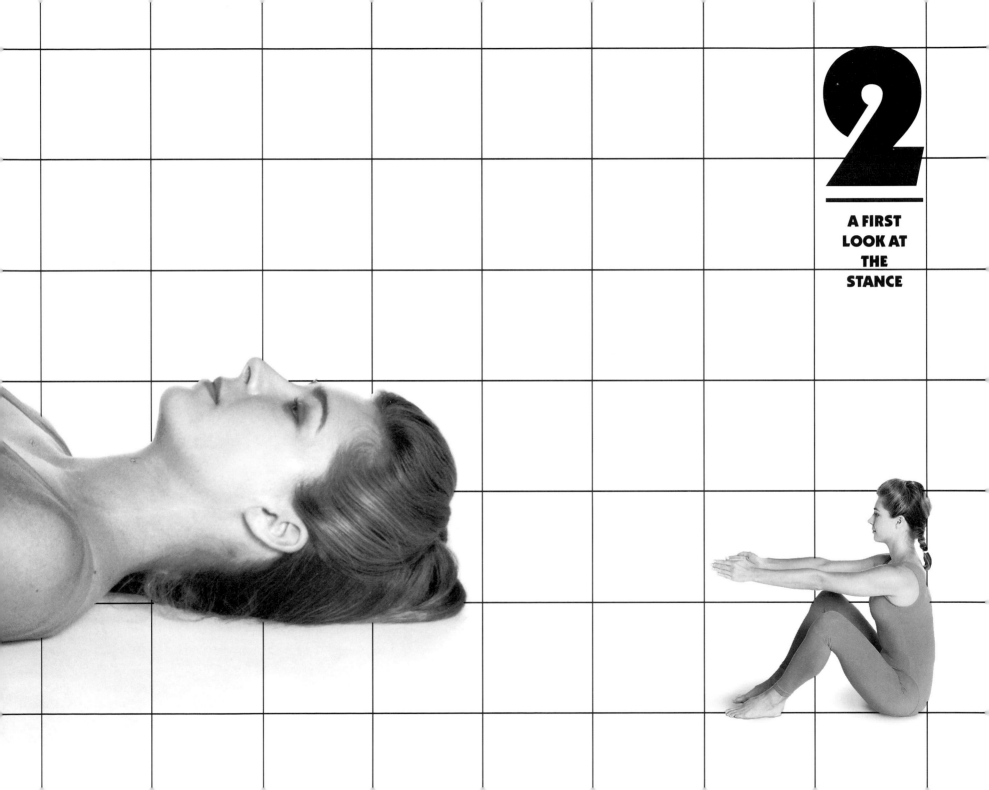

2

A FIRST LOOK AT THE STANCE

CHAPTER TWO

A FIRST LOOK AT THE STANCE

From our earliest childhood, people have been telling us to "stand up straight," but nobody seems to be able to tell us how. Usually we respond by assuming a stiff, rigid posture, knees locked even tighter and chest sticking way out so that the back is painfully arched. Even the most earnest of soldiers would find it difficult to maintain this posture for long, and certainly it's a far cry from what Mother Nature intended for us.

The Stance will tell you, for the first time, what standing up straight really means. We've already defined the ideal posture as Balanced Alignment, a state of skeletal and muscular balance in which gravity exerts no uneven pressure on the body—in which, in fact, gravity acts not as a downward drag but as an uplifting force. This state of balance is achieved through the Stance, which opens the joints from ankle to neck so that each body part is positioned directly above the one below. This is the ideal way for the body to situate itself in space, in its maximum length out from the center, since it causes the least friction and stress and makes the most efficient use of our energy.

The Stance will also:

- Erase the effects of previous habits of misalignment and the painful restrictions on your freedom of movement;

- Place your body in its ideal relationship with gravity, in which gravity acts as a support and not as an antagonist;

- Balance the action of opposing muscles, releasing tight ones and strengthening slack ones, so that each of your skeletal muscles is doing the job it was designed to do;

- Program your mind and body for the new, correct way of maintaining yourself in space.

The Stance will introduce you to a new concept and a new experience of gravity. Using a set of lively images to stimulate you in making the change from your old habitual way of standing to the new balanced way, it offers you an innovative way of *thinking* about your body in space, a new way of *being* in gravity, of situating yourself in the energy stream defined in Chapter One. From now on, whenever you choose to perceive consciously exactly where you are in space, you'll have a choice. The Stance grid provides an objective standard against which to measure yourself, a tool with which to *know* whether or not you're standing straight, in Balanced Alignment, and if not, how to get there.

By nature, we are symmetrical animals. We are bipeds, balanced evenly on two feet. Our arms and legs normally hang evenly on either side of the spine. The waist should be exactly level, front to back, as it bisects the torso. The spine should be exactly upright, its natural curves as long and shallow as possible, with the head resting easily at the top of the erect spine. The feet are designed to work best when parallel, with the toes pointing straight ahead.

This precise new placement of the parts of the body stacked correctly makes possible the state of Balanced Alignment, which in turn places us in the ideal relationship to gravity. Beginning at the feet and moving upward, the Stance will position you along the most powerful line of the energy stream, which is always potentially moving in and through your body, carrying you with its force—provided you don't interfere with it by blocking or locking. You'll learn how to call upon it at its strongest and most supportive, so that it carries you up as effortlessly as possible.

In the next chapter, we will observe your present way of standing, noticing where you've had problems and pain in the past. We will assess, part by part, where you're out of alignment in your habitual posture. Then we'll go through the Stance in detail, giving you the experience of correcting the sources of misalignment. For now, we'll go through the Stance in a general overview, so that you'll know what it looks and feels like.

Let's start with the most important basic principle of the Stance: *It is what we do below the hips that determines the balance, freedom and power of the body above the hips.* In other words, misalignment of the feet, knees and hips directly influences pain in the lower back, upper back and neck. The foundation of Balanced Alignment lies right *at* the foundation, at the base of support: the relation of foot to ankle, and of ankle to knee.

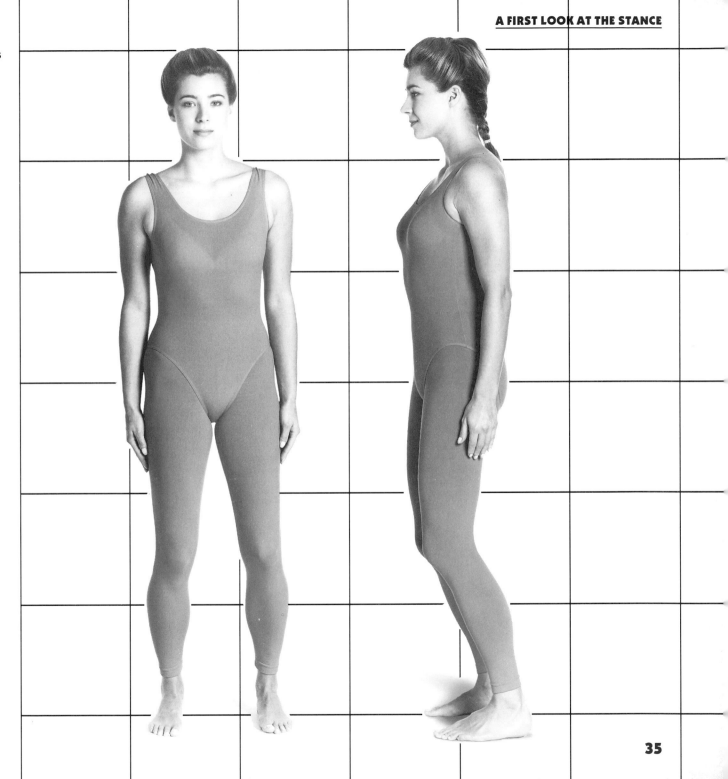

A look at the Stance, from the front and in profile, shows each part of the body lined up on a grid.

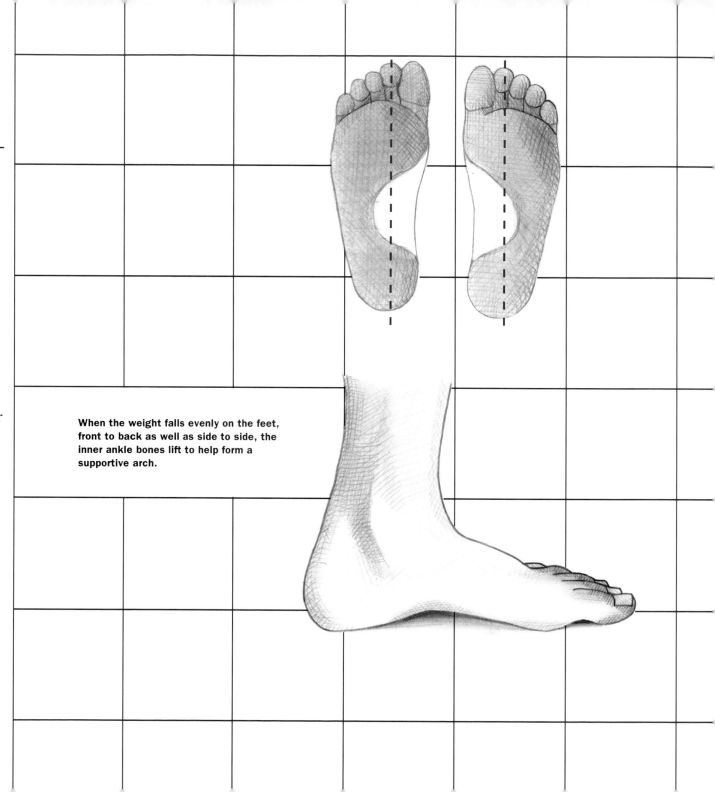

THE FEET

The feet are like two small platforms that provide your entire base of support. Given the height of your body, this is all the more reason for a precisely accurate placement of the feet.

In the Stance, your feet point straight ahead, their weight centered directly on a straight line running from the base of the second toe (the one next to the big toe) back through the center of the heel. The weight of your body should fall directly on the entire foot, not just on the heel or toes. As you'll learn in the next chapter, if your feet are the slightest bit out of alignment, the effect is unavoidable and you pay heavily for it farther up.

When the weight falls evenly on the feet, front to back as well as side to side, the inner ankle bones lift to help form a supportive arch.

THE STANCE

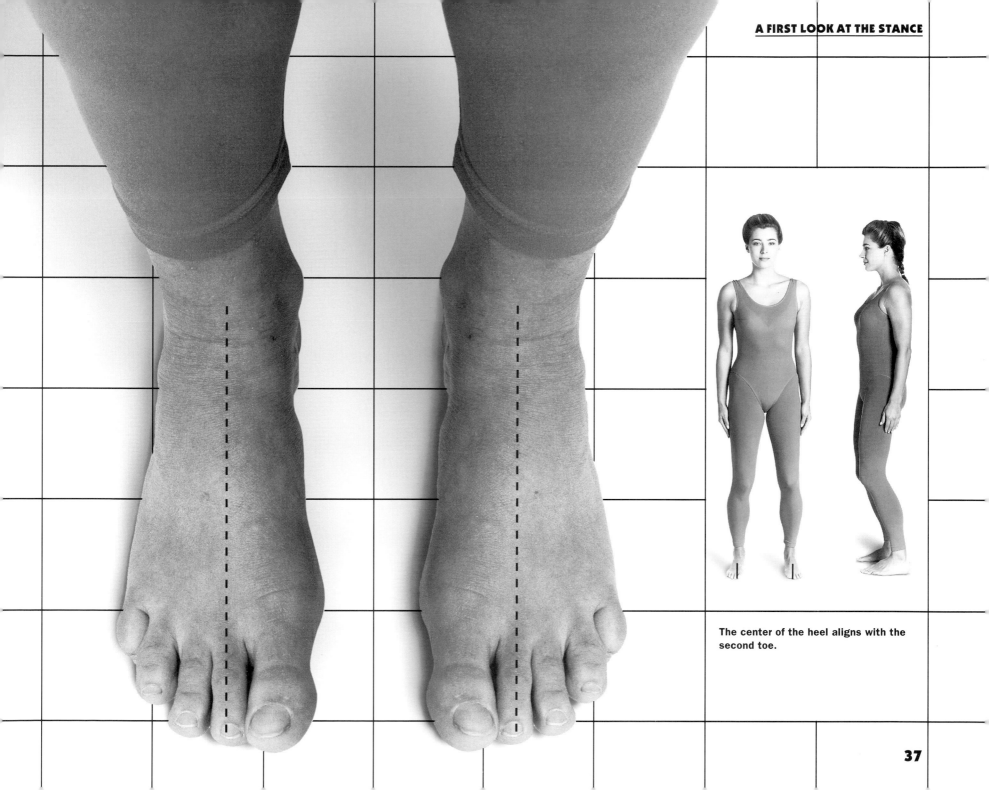

The center of the heel aligns with the second toe.

THE ANKLES

At right angles to the straight line passing through the center of the foot is the horizontal line of the ankle bones. This line, running through the ankle bones from side to side, must be *precisely* horizontal, tilted neither toward the insides nor the outsides of the feet.

Alignment of the feet and ankles is the basic element of the grid that establishes the foundation for the entire alignment of your body in space. It makes possible the full, free articulation of the ankle joint, the most important joint in the body, and allows you to flex (bend) forward at the ankle at a sharp angle to the foot—the most important first step in correcting your alignment. Many people can scarcely bend at their ankles at all, largely because this full flexion is interfered with by faulty ankle-foot alignment.

Imagine a RUBBER BAND running around the outside of both ankles, over the outer ankle bones. Tension must be maintained in the band by rolling the ankles slightly outward. This light tension is necessary to maintain the new position, in which the balance of each foot is centered over the line running from the second toe to the heel. It is the thought of aligning your foot along this center line *and* of lifting your inner ankle bone, simultaneously, that precisely aligns your foot.

The image of two FELT-TIPPED MARKERS growing out of the inner ankle bones, parallel to the floor, is also helpful in learning the Stance. If the ankles are rolled in, the imaginary pens will droop down and make black marks on the floor.

This seemingly small adjustment of the ankles, as

The ankle is the most important joint in your body —and the most underused.

you will see, engages muscles throughout the entire foot, leg and hip. I cannot emphasize strongly enough that very, very small shifts of weight in the ankle and foot, from just a little off-center to precisely on center, greatly affect the alignment of the entire body. From this new, firm foundation, the knees can bend as they were designed to: straight ahead, front to back. If the feet are not straight during the forward motion of walking (or running, or skating), the knees are torqued at every step, twisted like wrung-out washcloths. That is, the misaligned feet misdirect the knees, which are wrenched from side to side, strained by a sideways wobble they were never meant to have. This is a principal reason for the frequency of injury to the knees: as the link between foot and hip, the complex and sensitive knee joint is often the first to give way under stress. And the twisting of the knee joint literally arises out of a misaligned foot and ankle.

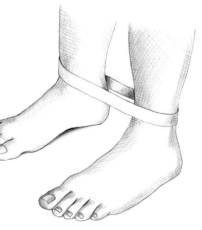

Maintain tension in the ELASTIC BAND by rolling the ankle bones to the outside.

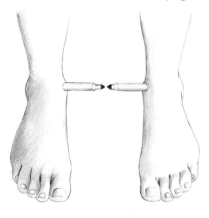

Lift the insides of the ankles to keep the FELT-TIPPED MARKERS from drooping.

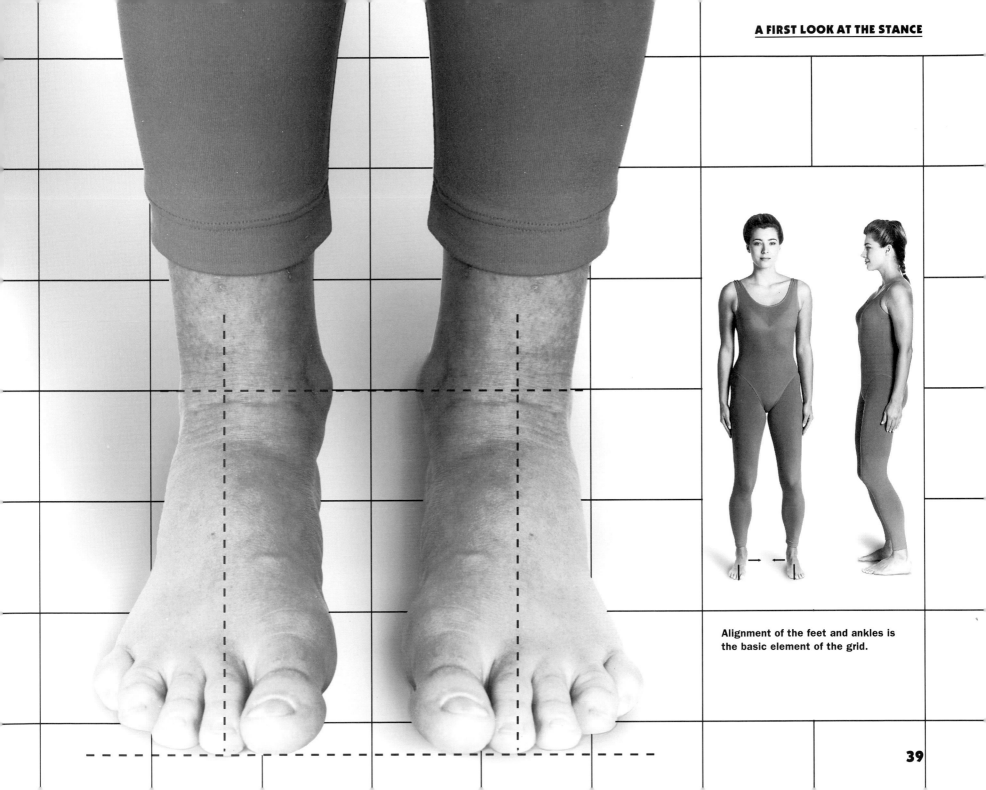

Alignment of the feet and ankles is the basic element of the grid.

THE KNEES

In the Stance, the knees are bent and the kneecaps point *straight ahead* like the two HEADLIGHTS of a car. Bending the knees and aiming them straight ahead releases the small of the back, lengthening the curve there (in the lumbar region, where the spine normally curves inward, just above the buttocks).

To check that the bend in the knees is deep enough, we'll use the image of HARPOONS, or spear guns, dangling straight down from each knee so that their tips meet the floor just in front of the second toe. At the same time, the heels remain firmly planted on the floor. Keeping the heels down while the knees bend at a sharp angle, with calves forward of the heels, stretches the Achilles tendons—and also drives the tips of the HARPOONS into the floor.

Alignment of the feet, ankles and knees is the foundation— the support—for everything that will happen above the knees. Feet and lower legs aim straight forward. This precise alignment of knees, ankles and feet automatically releases some of the pressure in the back that tips

BLOCKING THE FLOW

Locking the knees not only blocks the energy stream but also cuts off feeling from the feet, preventing you from experiencing your body as an integrated whole. The feet become incidental appendages, and this in turn immobilizes the ankle joint.

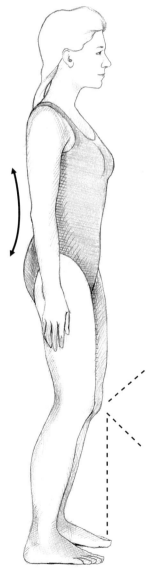

the pelvis forward, pushes the belly out and increases the curve in the lower back, compressing the vertebrae of the spine. The next step is to release this pressure still further.

Unlocking the knees repositions the pelvis and releases tightness in the lower back.

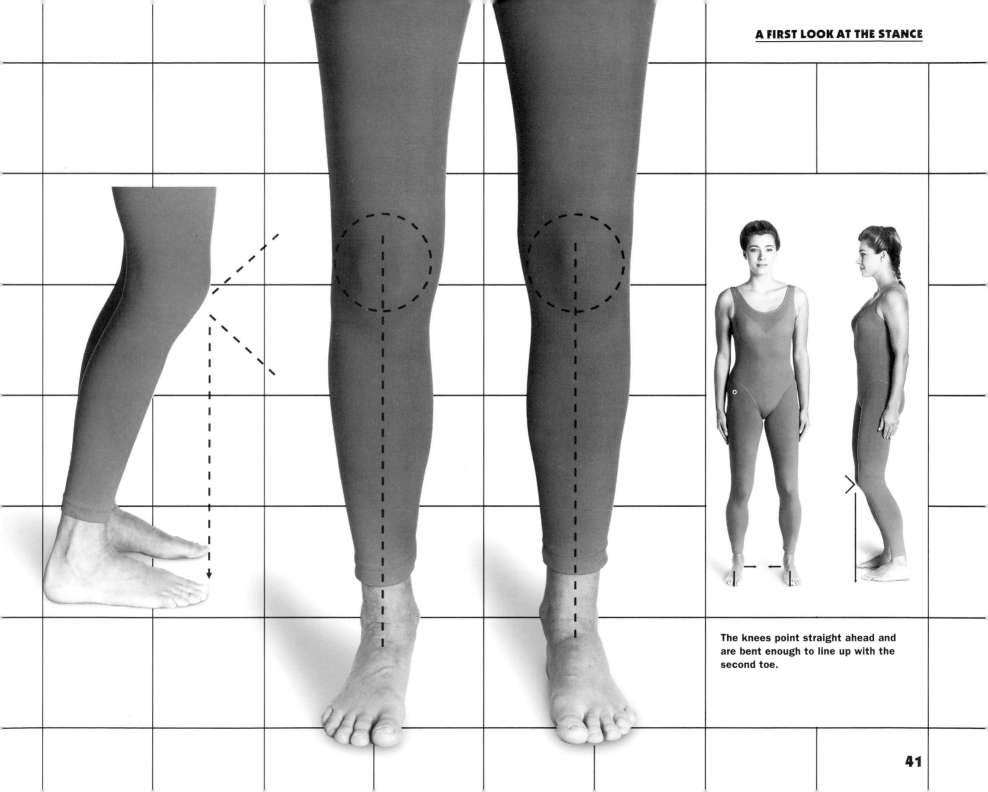

The knees point straight ahead and are bent enough to line up with the second toe.

THE PELVIS

The image of a sleepy raccoon living inside your pelvis at the tops of your legs, where they join your hips, will help you achieve more length in your lower back. (Some of these images may sound a little weird, but I promise they work!) The raccoon's eyes, one at each hip joint, are looking out. If the eyes are half closed, your hip joints are too flexed, too closed. To open the RACCOON EYES, you'll widen the angle between the tops of your thighs and your pelvis by thinking of lengthening your spine, so that your upper body rises more erectly up from your legs. At the same time, your knees and ankles are still very bent—an apparent paradox that will become clear as we go on.

As your lower back lengthens, its curve will become shallower, allowing your belly to flatten back against your spine instead of sagging forward. The more *space* there is between the surfaces of your joints, including each vertebra of your spine, the

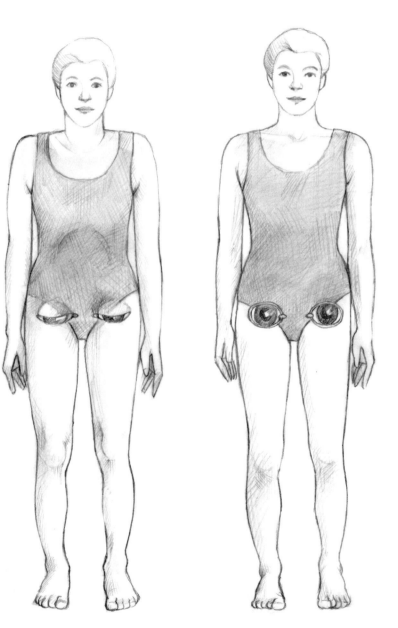

more *length* you'll have overall in your body.

The entire area from feet to hips should form a giant letter "H." The knees are at either end of the crosspiece of the letter, the thighs are the tops of the support pieces, and the ankles are the bottoms. For your legs to form the sides of the letter, perfectly parallel to each other, you'll have to think of *widening* your hips so that the hip bones are farther apart. You may feel that wider hips are the last thing you need; however, when you increase the distance between the *bones* in your hips so that your legs can line up, you have to contract the muscles in order to make your legs move apart, and this makes your thighs and hips actually appear trimmer!

Thinking in terms of lengthening the spine helps to widen the angle between the thighs and the pelvis.

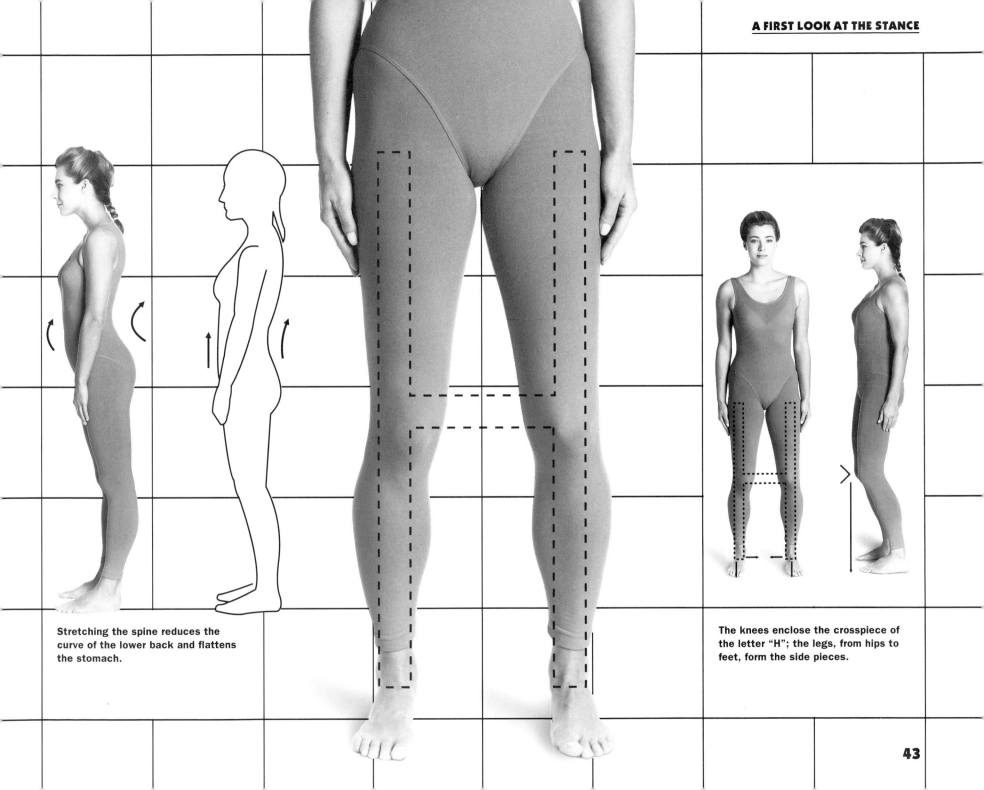

Stretching the spine reduces the curve of the lower back and flattens the stomach.

The knees enclose the crosspiece of the letter "H"; the legs, from hips to feet, form the side pieces.

THE TWO-WAY ENERGY STREAM

After aligning the lower half of your body, you can think of yourself as a TALL TREE. You have roots extending deep down into the earth, anchoring you firmly and giving you the support you need to grow tall. You also have sap running up through you, lifting your trunk high. Both these *opposing directional energies* are necessary if you are to grow tall and strong.

Like the tree, your body needs anchoring and lifting to situate itself effortlessly along the flow of gravity. The "sap" (your energy) must flow both down into your feet and up into and beyond your head.

An exit path. Once the lower half of your body has been stretched and the ankle, knee and hip joints are flexible and open, previously locked-in energy is free to flow. You can think of letting your weight drop down from your waist into your bent knees and open ankles. There is now an exit path for energy that may have been blocked in your back or hips. Your feet were meant to receive your weight and send it on down through into the ground like roots, holding you secure. This is achieved ideally, with the least effort and in perfect balanced alignment, when a plumbline dropped from the end of your bent knee will meet the floor just at the end of your second toe *and* when the center of your hip joint and the center of your foot are in a straight line. It's amazing how great an effect such a slight shift of weight forward, from back in the heels to the center of the feet, can have on the distribution of weight throughout the body.

This new placement of your body, farther forward than it used to be, and more lifted, will give you a strong sense of your torso and head being carried up on the rising energy stream. This doesn't mean that you lean or bend forward; rather, it's a forward *placement,* starting at the foot and ankle, and projecting up in a line through the top of your head.

Step and lift. In such a placement, looking from the side, the energy stream bisects the foot, right in the center of the arch, then continues up through the center of the knee, in its new, more bent position, up through the pelvis, continuing up straight through the torso, lifting the chest, through the middle of the neck and bisecting the head at the ear. And this magical placement of power and strength begins with a shift of the weight on the feet to a much more forward position.

Now, instead of locking joints and bones, like stilts, you have a line of energy that flows all the way up from the feet through the head while you press down, from the hips, through the knees, into the feet and down through them into the ground.

Our energy flows *down* from the waist, pressing down out of the hips, through the knees and ankles, down into and through the feet. At the same time, there is a steady stream, like a shaft of light, that flows *up*, from the feet through the knees, through the hips, through the center of the body up the spine, through the neck, into the head.

This two-way stream of energy is always present and available to your body; all you have to do is step into it and let it lift you up. This energy is also *dynamic*—as long as it's not interfered with, suppressed, or blocked by tightness that stiffens the body.

Easy balance. So, just as fixing and locking proceeds serially, in a wavelike pattern

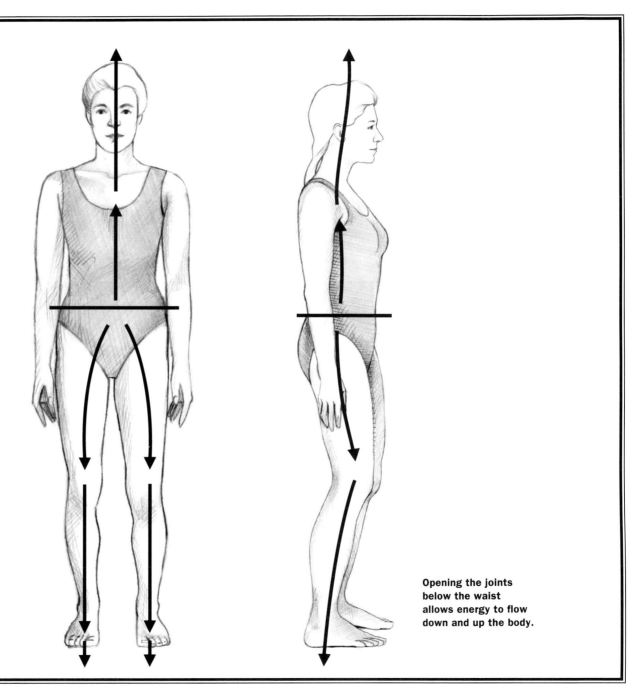

up the body, the restoration of true balance requires a sequential releasing down *as well as* a leaning into and lifting *up* by this beacon-like force. This goes all the way up *and* down the body, out the top of the head and down through the feet into the ground.

This, then, is the foundation of Balanced Alignment. When the relationship of foot to ankle and ankle to knee is correct, when the weight falls centered onto the foot, which happens when the knee is pressed forward and the ankle is free to flex so that a plumbline would fall from the kneecap to the center of the foot, just behind the toes—then the rest of the body can balance lightly and easily above this flexible yet very secure foundation.

Remember, *it is what we do below the hip that determines our ease and balance above it.*

Opening the joints below the waist allows energy to flow down and up the body.

THE WAIST

Keeping the correct alignment of feet, ankles, knees and hips in mind, think of your pelvis and buttocks, from front to back, as a PAIL OF WATER. The top of your hips forms the rim of the pail, which is parallel to the ground and level from front to back so that the water inside stays level. If you stand with your pelvis tipped forward and your belly pushed out, the water in the pail will pour out the front because the pail is tilted forward. To keep the water from spilling, you'll have to draw in your abdominal muscles, which will also flatten the small of your back.

The connection between the abdomen and the back is a close and vital one because their muscles work together to support the column of the spine. If either one sags forward because of weak muscles and/or improper alignment, the spine is pulled too far forward in the small of the back. The spine curves there naturally, but it should form only a slight curve—not the short, deep one that occurs without proper support. Merely by thinking of lengthening your lower torso between your hips and your waist *upward* and keeping your PAIL OF WATER level, you'll be able to change the shape of your midsection from thick and formless to defined and slender.

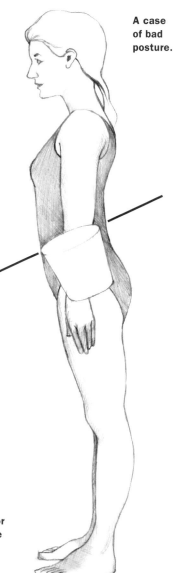

A case of bad posture.

Weak stomach and/or back muscles pull the lower spine forward, causing swayback.

46

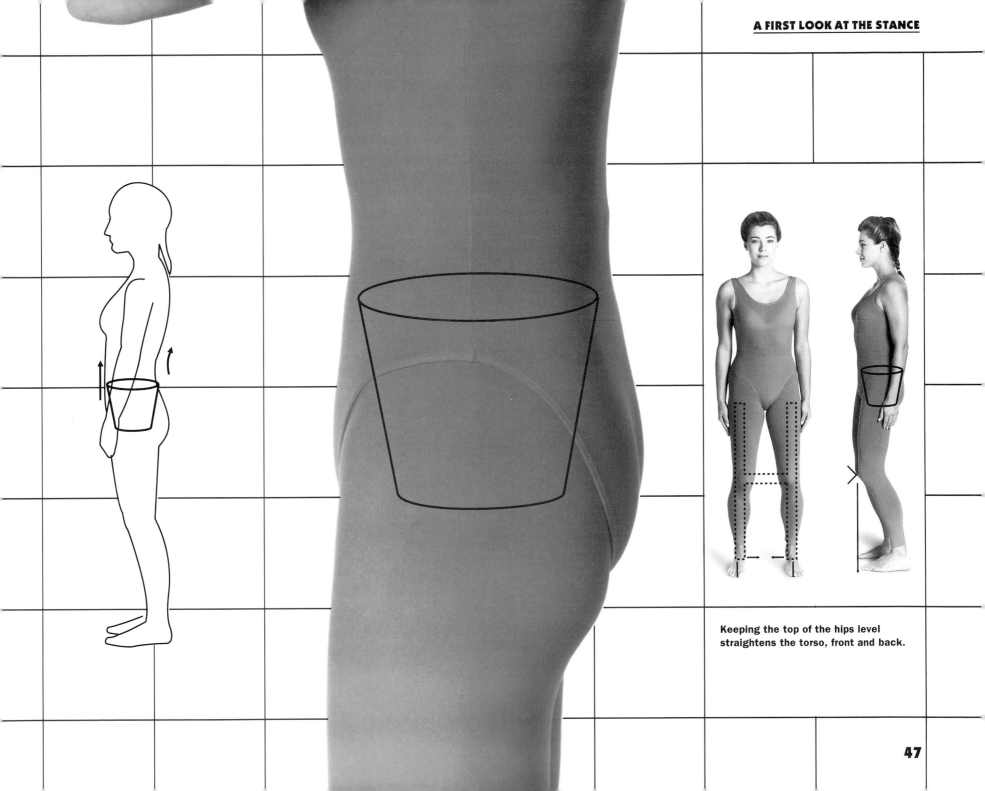

Keeping the top of the hips level
straightens the torso, front and back.

47

THE SPINE

THE STANCE

Only at its maximum extension does the spine move successfully and easily as a unit instead of bending and collapsing. Imagine inserting SHIMS, little wedges of wood, between your hip bones and your bottom ribs. Gradually add another, and another, continuing to become taller by increasing the distance between hips and ribs. You are creating this space for the SHIMS by lengthening your spine *from within*.

When your spine is aligned over your feet in the precise relationship of the Stance, you'll be substituting *alignment* for *effort* and releasing blocked energy—the energy that before

Length, length, and more length.

was lost through locking the knees and the downward pressure of the torso sinking. Through repetitions, these small acts of conscious alignment will become second nature, especially when you've begun to experience the ease, power and pleasure of

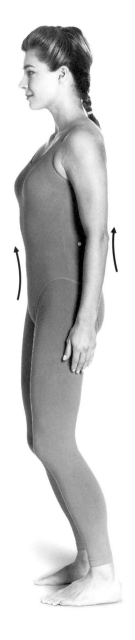

your whole body moving fluidly along on the gravity stream.

When you lengthen your spine by thinking of inserting the SHIMS, one by one, you'll continue the lengthening and flattening of the abdominal muscles and the lengthening of the lower back muscles that began with the leveling of the PAIL OF WATER. This will continue the narrowing from front to back of your whole torso, from hips upward, that places you in the most precise and effective alignment on that upward-flowing stream.

As the abdomen and lower back straighten, the torso falls into alignment over the ankles and feet.

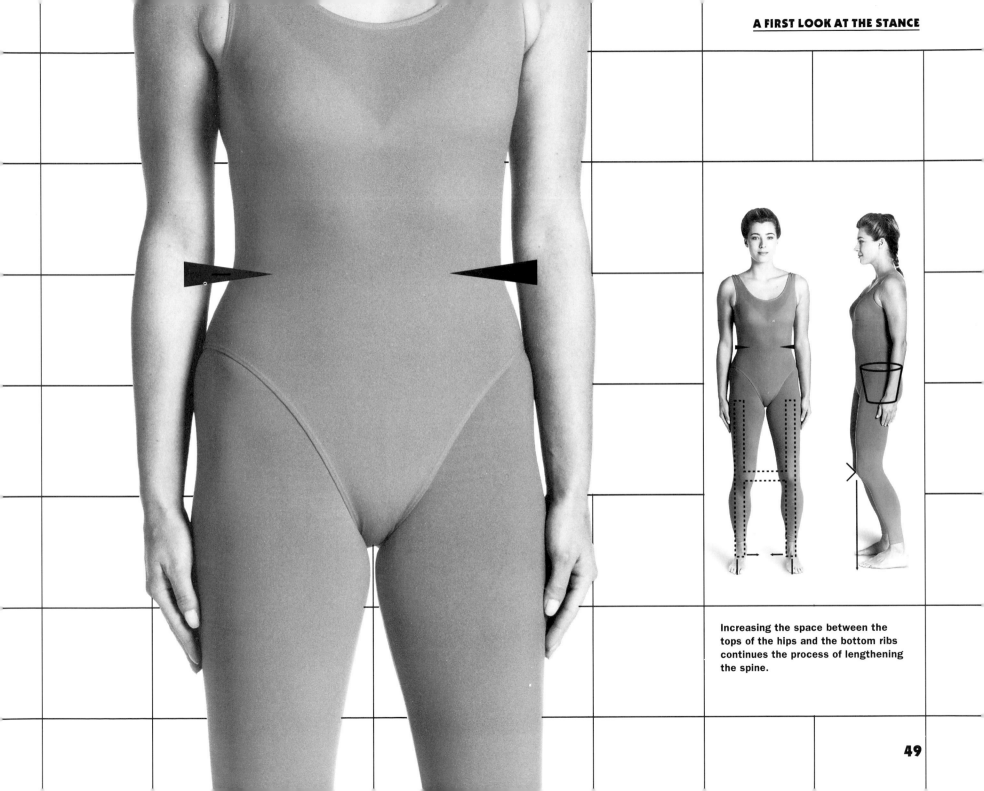

Increasing the space between the
tops of the hips and the bottom ribs
continues the process of lengthening
the spine.

THE CHEST

Now we come to another weird but very effective image. Picture a PLUNGER, or plumber's helper, stuck to the middle of your chest, its long handle sticking straight out parallel to the floor. To keep the handle from drooping down toward the ground, you must lengthen your upper torso without becoming swaybacked. Your chest should not slump forward, collapsed by your shoulders pulling forward, nor should it arch back, military style, pulled up and stiff.

In the Stance, your upper body will be long and straight, aiming straight ahead like your feet, knees and hips.

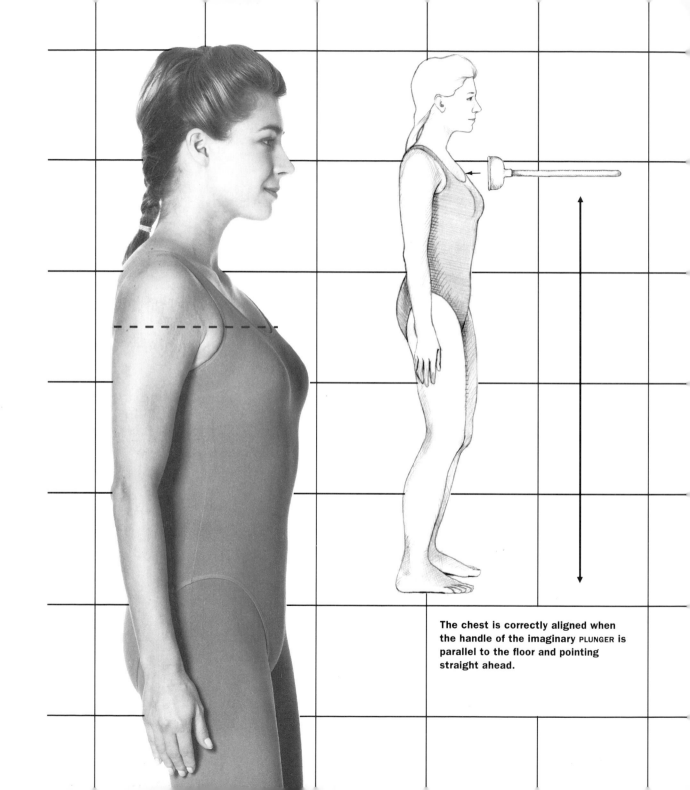

The chest is correctly aligned when the handle of the imaginary PLUNGER is parallel to the floor and pointing straight ahead.

THE SHOULDERS

In proper alignment, the shoulders must be perfectly straight across, above an erect back and upper chest. Imagine an old-fashioned milkmaid, carrying her pails of milk at either end of a yoke extending across her upper back. To keep the pails from spilling, she must keep her shoulders very level, down and wide. If she bends backwards, the weight of the pails will be too heavy; forward, and they'll pull her over.

With the image of the MILKMAID'S YOKE, the Stance adds a horizontal dimension as you think your shoulders *wide,* opening them up in a line extending out to each side.

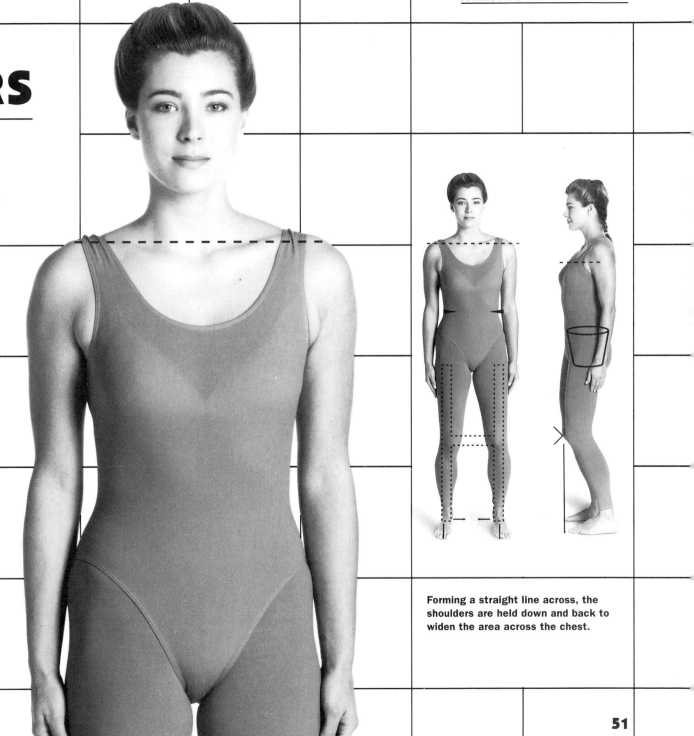

Forming a straight line across, the shoulders are held down and back to widen the area across the chest.

THE NECK

The longer the neck, the more *precisely balanced* the head. And the more balanced the head, the more *effortlessly* it poises upon the neck, floating on the rising stream of energy. It always amazes me that when my head is lightly balanced as high as possible above my hips, I have the *least* feeling of effort. The higher and longer, the easier.

Thinking of your neck as an ACCORDION, stretching longer and longer, will help position your head so that it lines straight up out of your shoulders.

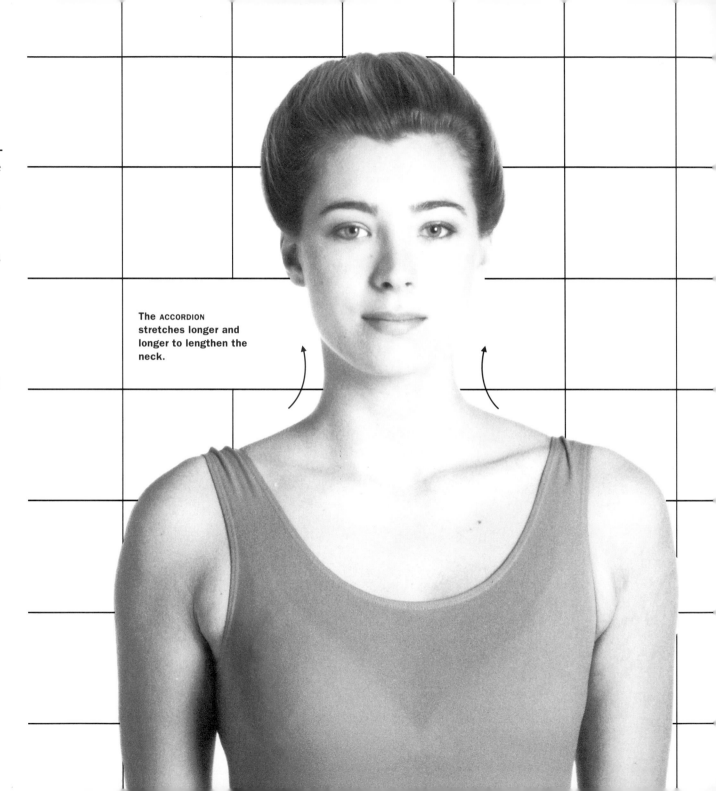

The ACCORDION stretches longer and longer to lengthen the neck.

THE HEAD

The last image we'll use in the Stance is that of a GOLDEN HOOK fastened to the top of your head. Its purpose is to affix your body to an imaginary beam or ceiling above so that you can hang from it, relaxed, as a skeleton hangs from a pole in an anatomy classroom. Just think yourself *tall* enough to allow the hook to reach its eye in the ceiling—then let go, letting yourself hang freely from it.

Thinking of the GOLDEN HOOK will keep your upper-body alignment straight. This crucial alignment prevents the bowing and upper-body slump that is a particular problem for people who sit at desks all day or do any kind of prolonged close work: their shoulders tend to fall forward, with the head projecting horizontally into space, which compresses the spine and the entire torso. This lengthening also helps to reverse the shortening of the spine that is associated with aging and that is neither inevitable nor even normal, but a correctable habit.

Think tall! The GOLDEN HOOK will find its way to the eye as you complete the stretch of the Stance.

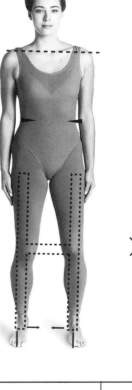

ALL THE WAY UP

To lift your spine still further, imagine standing in a gale-force wind with an important PIECE OF PAPER under your heels. If you press down from inside the Achilles tendons running up the backs of your heels and lengthen your spine as you exert this pressure downward, you can keep the paper from blowing away. This action anchors you in your feet and sends a subtle message to your spine that it's safe to stretch out to its full length.

THE VANCE STANCE

The Stance is a standard to which we'll keep referring throughout this book; it should become the basis for everything you do, every move you make—your whole bodily relationship to the world. Eventually, you'll be able to run through it in just a few seconds, joint by joint, image by image, almost automatically, and it will become a resource to call upon throughout your day, a rapid, systematic release of tension that restores ease and fluidity to all your movement.

To sum up: The Stance opens the joints and muscles, from ankles to neck, so that each body part is positioned quite precisely above the one below. This

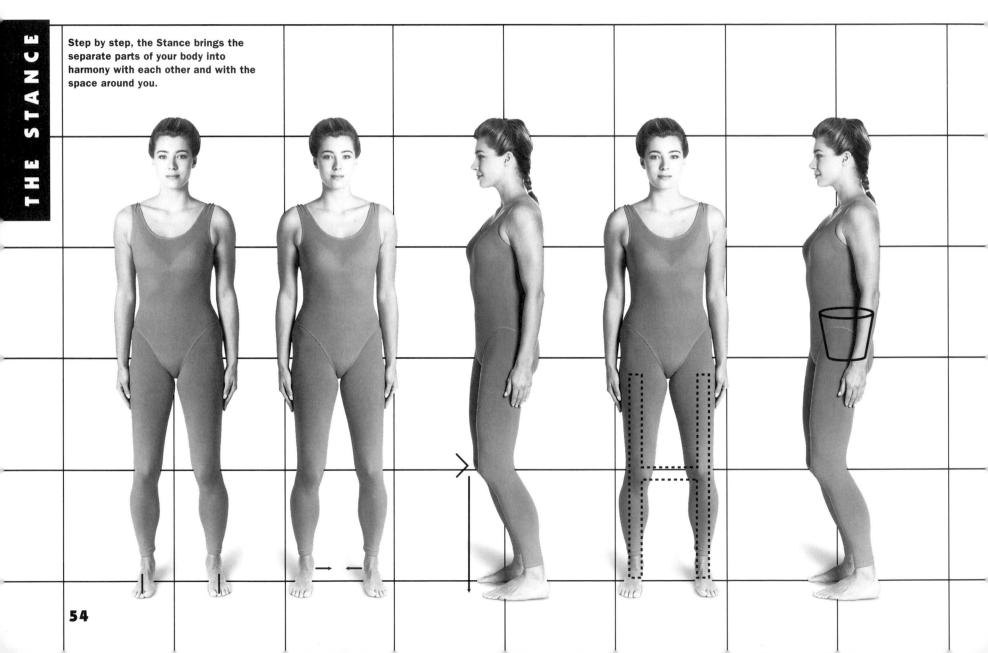

THE STANCE

Step by step, the Stance brings the separate parts of your body into harmony with each other and with the space around you.

encourages you to extend your body in all directions to feel maximum length, which is the ideal way for the body to situate itself in space. This causes the

least stress, and makes the most efficient use of your energy.

Now you know how to stand up straight—intellectually, at least. You've been introduced to

a new way of feeling where you are in space and how your body is aligned. The Stance gives you a grid, an objective measure on which to experience yourself

in Balanced Alignment. In the next chapter, we'll go through each step of the Stance, image by image, and see how you personally measure up.

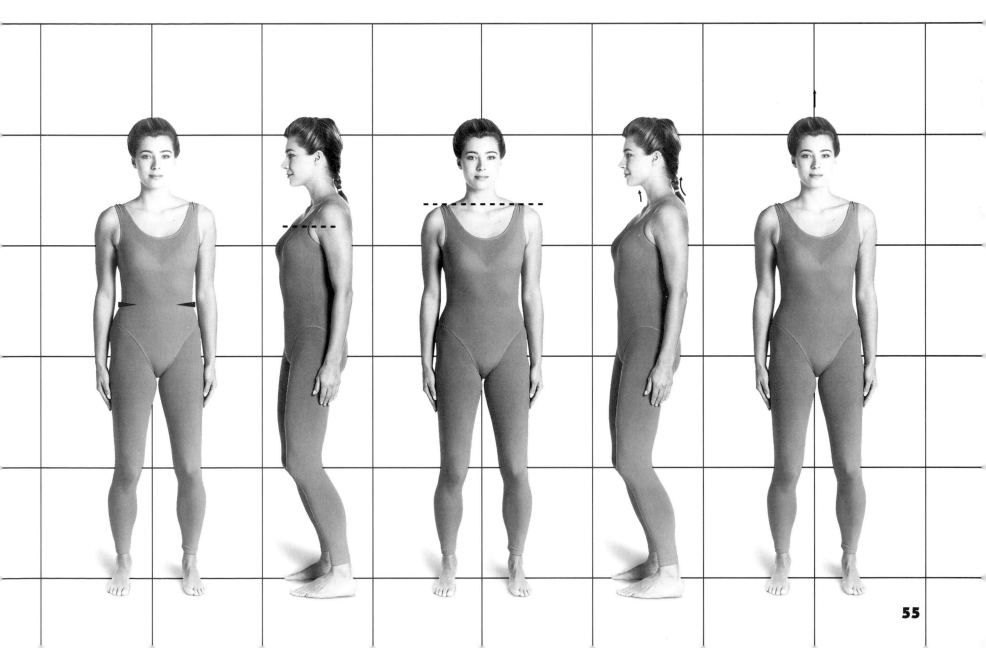

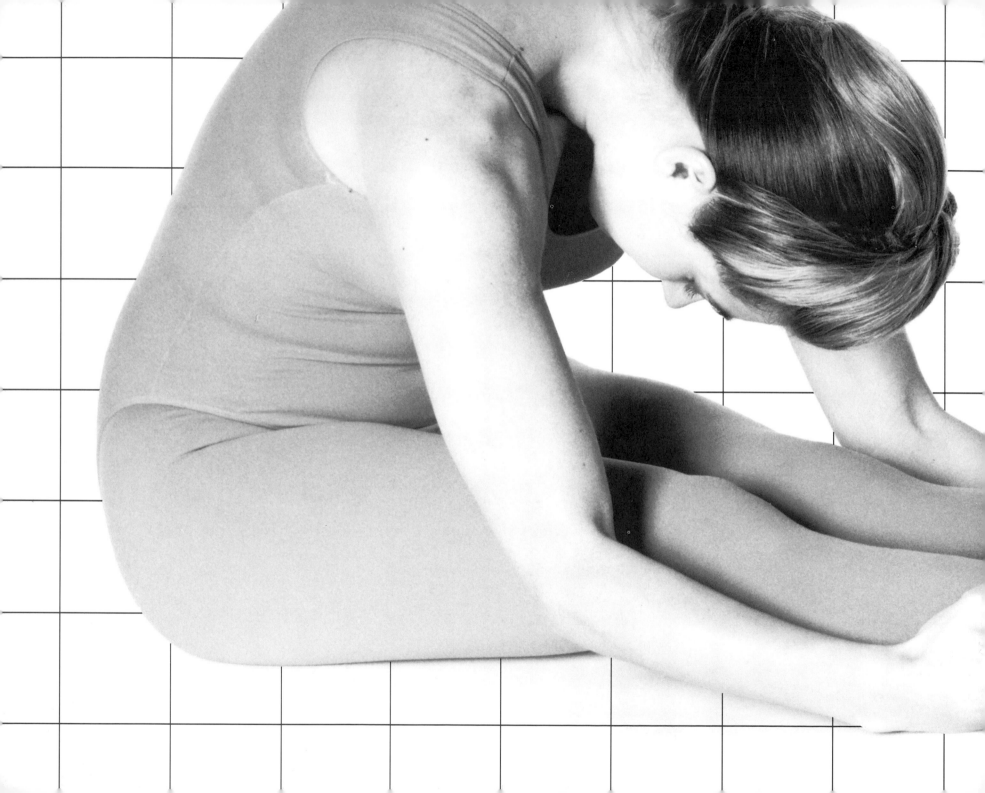

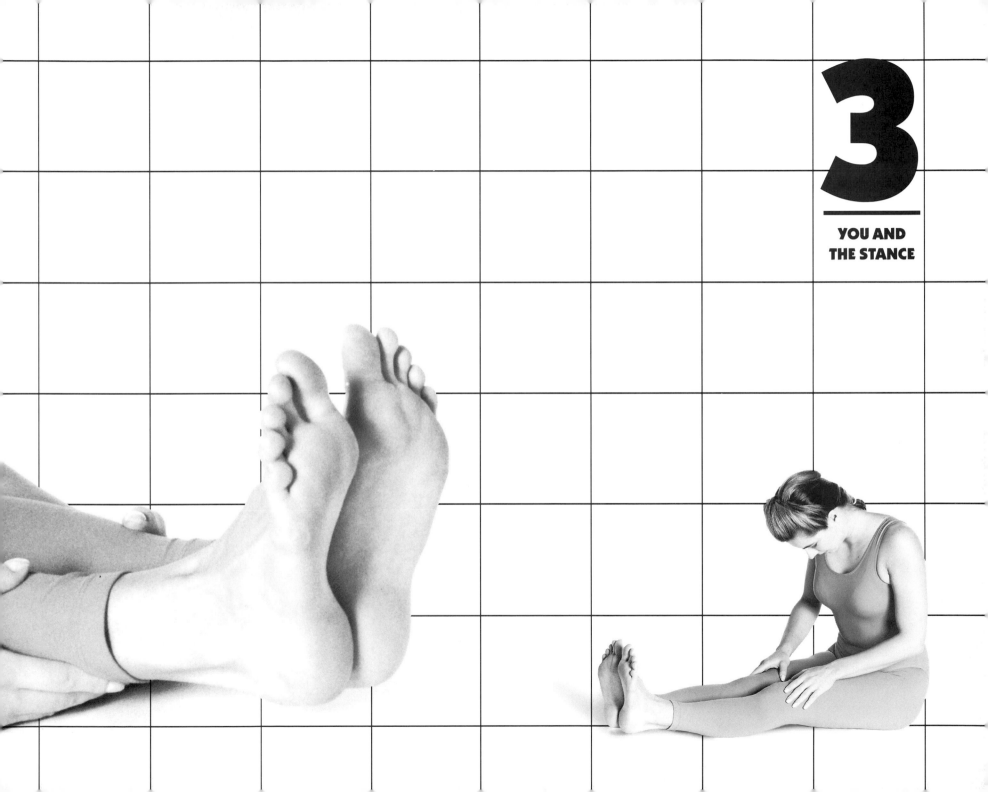

CHAPTER THREE

YOU AND THE STANCE

Before we can expect you to be able to do the Stance, we have to find out precisely how you stand right now. Your mind needs to understand the exact degrees of difference between the *ideal* we now have of the Stance and the *reality* of how you are at this moment. These discrepancies will tell us where to begin work, to bring you to a new, higher level. We will then assume the Stance, beginning with the feet and ankles and working our way up through the whole body so that you can begin to experience the freedom of Balanced Alignment.

First, as a reminder, turn your attention to the list of images at the right. These will be our points of reference when we take the Stance later on in this chapter.

THE STANCE IN BRIEF

- **FELT-TIPPED PENS**

  Ankles parallel to the floor, feet pointing straight ahead.

- **ELASTIC BAND**

  Ankles maintaining sufficient tension to lift arches.

- **HEADLIGHTS**

  Knees pointing straight ahead.

- **HARPOONS**

  Knees and ankles hinged to bring knees into alignment over ends of toes.

- **RACCOON EYES**

  Hip joints in front released and open so that the "eyes" are opened wide and looking straight out, not half-closed (as when the hip joints are partially flexed).

- **PAIL OF WATER**

  Waistline level, parallel with the ground, tipped neither forward or back nor side to side.

- **SHIMS**

  Space added between hips and ribs to lengthen the torso up out of the pelvis.

- **PLUNGER**

  Chest erect and wide, not stooped or collapsed, so that the plunger handle sticks straight out in front rather than drooping down toward the floor.

- **MILKMAID'S YOKE**

  Shoulders parallel and easily dropped down and back, allowing the "milk pails" to hang comfortably on either side.

- **ACCORDION**

  Neck long, lining up the head as it rises straight up from the shoulders.

- **GOLDEN HOOK**

  The whole body suspended, tall and easy, from the "eye" overhead.

- **PIECE OF PAPER**

  Heels pressed down as a counterforce to the lift of the torso; energy pressing down from the hips into the heels and flowing equally up out of the waist, lengthening the spine all the way up through the top of the head.

IDENTIFYING THE "TROUBLE SPOTS"

Your present way of standing reflects your whole life history of bodily injuries and the accumulated effects of bad postural habits. We will go through your body, part by part, assessing what is crooked, unsymmetrical and painful, and noting as well any past injuries and current problem areas.

Old habits of imbalance that cause uneven pressure, stress that you may be experiencing in your present activity, damage from weaknesses or injuries that may have long since sunk below the threshold of consciousness— all will be brought into awareness, recognized and corrected.

Keep in mind that as a child you could well have imitated compensations adopted by your parents—a foot turned out, or a shoulder carried higher on one side. You may have also copied the moves of peers or idols— a pigeon-toed walk or a rolling gait.

You'll become aware, too, of postural habits from your current daily life, "occupational hazards" that cause continual stress and interfere with your potential balanced relationship with

gravity: demanding and uneven weight-bearing (such as carrying heavy bags or a shoulder bag) or stressful occupations (standing at a counter all day, carrying heavy trays or heavy children, hunching over a computer or driving for long hours). The influence of habit and of any and all injuries upon your ability to stand straight can be surprisingly great.

Write down any injuries, severe illnesses or other traumas as we discover them, perhaps noting as well any emotions associated with them that may arise. Examples: "Around the age of eight, I was constantly twisting my ankles. I never felt secure on my feet." Or, "From about the age of fifteen, I couldn't run easily. My legs and feet felt uncoordinated with each other and with the rest of my body. I remember I had trouble keeping up in a game of dodgeball or soccer." What you remember from the past, even from very far back, may still be exerting an inhibiting influence on the way you use your body. This list will help you to see the inter-connectedness of your body and the way past injuries or habitual misuse may be contributing to pain you have now.

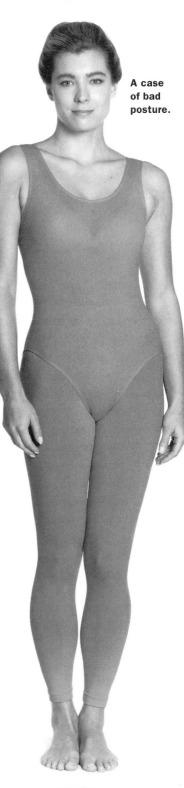

A case of bad posture.

STANDING

Let's begin our inventory to see where you are right now. To allow a full, frank view of your body, stand in front of a full-length mirror with few or (better) no clothes on. Leave your feet bare—no shoes, socks or footed tights. Don't try to make any adjustments yet; simply stand in your usual, old way, letting the real you "hang out." Keep your legs together at first so the ankle bones touch, as do the big-toe joints and optimally the insides of the knees.

Lower body, front view. The legs should touch lightly at the ankle and knee bones. If there is no contact anywhere from your ankles to your crotch, you have *bowlegs*. Bowlegs are commonly believed to result from crookedness of the leg bones (and to therefore be an orthopedic problem); however, in most cases they are caused simply by an incorrect positioning of the legs from ankles to hips, which in turn causes the knees to hyperextend (lock back) and bow outward because of the backward pressure.

The difference between your present way of standing and the Stance reflects your history of bodily injuries and/or the accumulation of bad postural habits.

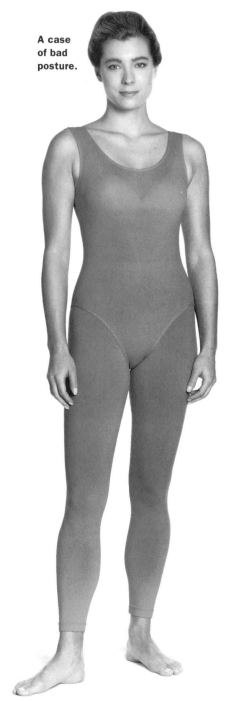

A case of bad posture.

If your knees overlap when your feet and ankles are together, you have *knock-knees.* (This condition often produces a small pouch of fat at the knee, even in very thin people, that does not respond to dieting or aerobic exercises.) An over-lapping of the thighs halfway between knee and crotch is also "knocking." A variation of this condition occurs when the thighs are too tight together, with the lower legs splayed apart.

When you have ascertained your leg shape, give a little jump and spread your feet to hip-width. Imagine that you're standing around bored, waiting in line for a bus or a bank teller, or biding your time at a dull cocktail party.

What do you notice about your reflection in the mirror? Look for signs of misalignment from your feet to your hips to your shoulders. Is one side more turned out or higher than the other? Are your hands level? As symmetrical beings, we are meant to be evenly balanced on our feet. When one element or joint is even slightly out of kilter, the effect is felt throughout the

Our feet were designed to work best when parallel to each other with the toes facing straight ahead. This allows the ankles to hinge properly, front to back.

body—as we'll see when we assume the Stance.

Take a close look at your feet and ankles—the base of support for the rest of your body. Do your feet turn out at an angle? (Most people's do. We seem to have developed this habit to give us more stability as toddlers.) Can you feel exactly where your weight falls on your feet? Is it the same on each foot? Is it the same front to back? Most likely your weight is settled back in your heels and toward the inner edges of your feet, rolling toward the inner ankle bones and the insides of the big toes. This position, called *pronation,* is the basis (in both senses of the word) of

Uneven weight distribution on the feet due to unbalanced alignment can result in bunions, calluses and hammertoes.

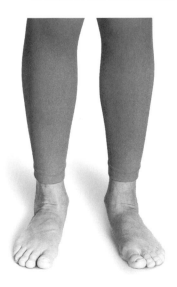

most structural problems higher up in the body. It results, first of all, in "fallen arches" or "flat feet." Devices such as arch supports and orthotics (custom-made foot supports) are designed to correct this, but they can't really do their job of supplying an arch until the feet are pointing straight ahead. (Consciously trying to lift the arch helps, and is part of our work, but it's impossible to do this effectively unless the feet are properly aligned.)

Write down what you've found out about your feet and legs, and about where you hold your weight. Most injuries to the ankle tend to result in some limitation of movement, which can almost always be corrected with appropriate exercises—provided you become aware of the limitation. Have you ever sprained an ankle? Stepped off a curb and wrenched an ankle? Broken an ankle, foot or toe? Have you ever, for any reason, limped for any length of time? Used crutches or a cane or wheelchair? It's astonishing how often—and how deep—we bury the memory of these events; but they can be retrieved if you direct your attention to them. Try to encourage every emotion and

60

memory connected with your body's history to rise to the surface and reveal itself, so that you can recognize any sloppy habits or compensations that account for your "normal" way of standing.

If you have bowlegs or knock-knees, you're likely to have knee troubles and probably pain. Except for direct-contact blows, most damage to the knee results from a previous weakening of the joint through misalignment of the ankles and hips, which makes it susceptible to a variety of stress injuries. In the war of misalignment, the first victim is often the knee joint. *Runner's knee* or *skier's knee* is usually caused by a misaligned knee being twisted and stressed beyond the expiration of its "grace period." The condition is made worse if the feet are splayed out to either side while the hips are more or less frontal. These two opposing forces meet at the knee, which is torqued in response to this twisting stress. The resulting damage and pain can be great, another demonstration of the vital importance of correct positioning of the feet and ankles.

Do you remember any injuries to your knees? Any twisting? Any

breaks, or tears in the cartilage? If you have bowlegs or knock-knees, be aware of just how far your knees deviate from aiming straight ahead. In the past, if

---

The locked-joint way of standing blocks the two-way flow of energy.

---

your feet were pointing sideways, your knees were forced to "decide" which way to go with every step. During the forward motion of walking (or running, or skating), the lower leg would be turned out at the bottom and the knee would be torqued. The occurrence of so many knee injuries bears this out.

Many people have had injuries in sports, especially men: a football tackle that brought them down too hard; a slide into home plate that caused a sharp, if transient, pain in the knee; turning too fast on the tennis court. Injuries such as these, even if far in the past, are not forgotten by the body.

Perhaps you've had surgery to repair one knee or both. Notice now if one leg looks and/or feels different from the other, and write that down. Later

we will explore ways of reducing the impact this disparity may be having on your life in the present.

Lower body, side view. Now turn sideways to the mirror and look again at your lower legs. Do your calves or the backs of your knees fall *behind* an imaginary line drawn straight up from your heels? If so, your knees are *hyperextended*—the joints are pushed too far back, perhaps as far back as they will extend, and locked in position. This means that the ankle, knee and hip joints are functioning not as a spring but as a stiff, rigid unit, which in turn means that neither the ankles nor the hips can hinge properly. Hyperextended knees virtually fuse the whole lower body, from feet to hips, so that every step you take is a jolt to the spine and you're vulnerable to almost every possible form of orthopedic injury. *Hyperextending (or just locking) your knees is the single most damaging thing you can do to your body.*

Hyperextending the knees affects the pelvis and the small of the back, moving the entire body out of the flow of gravity.

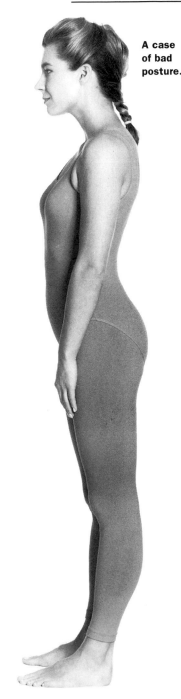

A case of bad posture.

Next, look at your buttocks. Do they stick out behind, making a little "shelf"? This is *swayback*. Does your abdomen stick out in front (no matter how many sit-ups you do)? This *potbelly* is related to swayback and to most back pain. Check to see if your waistline is level; with swayback, it will tilt toward the front.

Upper body. Still in profile, look at your torso. Does it slump down, collapsing into your waist? Or does it look extremely rounded? This is *"dowager's hump."* Does your neck look

It is vital to regain aware-ness of what you're doing with your body.

compressed, bringing your head too close to your shoulders? Are your shoulders rounded forward? Does your head jut forward? Recall incidents of lower-back pain, due to abdominal surgery, perhaps, or to a miscarriage.

Turn back now to face the mirror with your feet hip-width apart. Look at your waistline. Is one side higher than the other? Did you ever have a back injury on that side? Look at your midline, navel to neck. This vertical line may veer off-center due to *scoliosis*, or curvature of the spine, a condition long thought to be largely uncorrectable but that in fact responds quickly when worked on with stretching and strengthening exercises. Does one hand hang lower than the other, or are you carrying one arm and hand forward of the other? Uneven position of the hands also reveals symptoms of scoliosis. Check to see whether one side of your chest is more forward than the other. Do you have neck pain on that side?

Notice whether your chest tends to be somewhat caved in. Recall a blow to a breast, or surgery there, or a broken breast bone that may have taught you to hunch over in a protective compensation. Women often hunch because their breasts were the "wrong" size at the wrong time. Men sometimes choose a less aggressive posture, mistaking collapsing for a flexible, natural grace. Are you perhaps holding your chest stiffly

up and out so that your ribs are held fixed, permanently expanded? This is called *barrel chest* and is not as permanent a condition as it may seem. When we awaken other muscles that will permit you to let go in this area, your chest can relax and flatten all around your spine, restoring flexibility to your ribs.

Have you ever sustained a blow or fall—a direct hit in karate, a powerful check in ice hockey—that might have broken one or more ribs? Since the ribs enclose the breathing apparatus, working on this area can bring surprising improvement in breathing. I've had clients whose attacks of asthma were greatly relieved, sometimes entirely eliminated, after we worked through the chest and ribs.

Raised shoulders (or one shoulder carried higher than the other) cause tightening of the muscles in the back and neck.

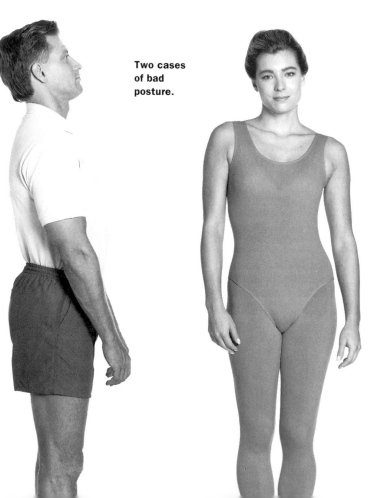

Two cases of bad posture.

Look at your shoulders. Are they level? Think back to a shoulder dislocation or broken collarbone. Are you holding one shoulder higher than the other? This is a habit frequently acquired when carrying shoulder bags, books, suitcases or any weight habitually on one side. (Doing this can also lead to carrying one hip higher than the other to counterbalance the weight above.)

Note carefully the precise alignment of your head over your neck. Do you tend to carry it to one side? Any habitual tilt or turn of the head off-center is frequently a source of *chronic neck pain*. Are your head and neck together lined up with the midline of your body? Is your head projected forward of your neck or tilted back on a neck that is arched too far forward?

One way to check the positioning of your head is to check your line of sight. Are you looking straight ahead, or up or down? Neck pain may be caused by having to keep turning your head in an effort to see straight in front of you. Sometimes this results from unequal strength of vision; the stronger eye dominates, so that the head keeps turning to bring that eye farther to the front. Or it may be the final product of misaligned feet or hips, or scoliosis. You may be looking straight ahead, but your body is turned.

Have you ever pulled a neck muscle in an accident or worn a neck brace for any length of time? Think back to a car accident, and whiplash, or even a slight slip in the rain. Perhaps you tend to turn your head to one side in order to favor a slightly deaf ear. Or perhaps you're unconsciously mimicking someone close to you.

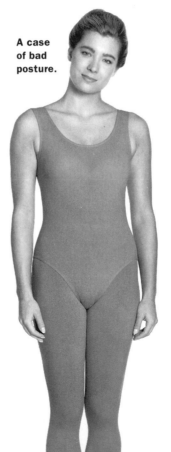

A case of bad posture.

Chronic neck pain can occur when the head is habitually held at an angle or off-center in relation to the midline of the body.

PAST INJURY, PRESENT PAIN

MARTHA'S STORY

The connection between a past injury and present pain was graphically demonstrated by Martha, a student in one of my classes, whose painful right hip had not responded to medical treatment or chiropractic care. When I asked her if she'd ever injured her right foot or ankle, she mentioned a bad fall some years back in which she had twisted her ankle severely and was unable to walk for two weeks. I proposed that the two were connected.

When we did the Thirty-Four Movements, it was obvious at once that for all these years she'd been holding her right hip high—originally in order to favor the injured ankle. The problem was that even after the ankle healed, she continued unconsciously to hold tension in the hip because the ankle had never been released properly after its trauma; that is, once it was healed, she'd never consciously worked to stretch the muscles that had been held immobile for so long. It was the hip that had begun to hurt in protest against the strain caused by improper alignment, so we had to work through the tightness in the ankle before we could address the hip problem.

"You know," Martha said, "I always *thought* there was a connection between my ankle and my hip. You've finally shown what I've always suspected but could never prove."

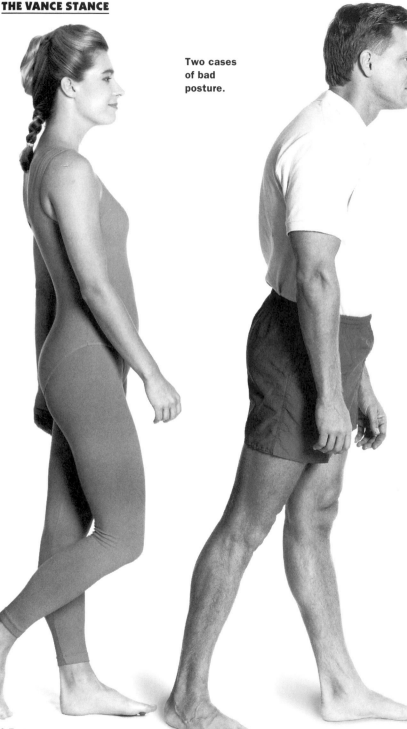

Two cases
of bad
posture.

WALKING

Now that we have a good idea of how you stand, let's look at how you walk. Stroll around the room. *Feel* how you do what you do. What makes your walk distinctive? Do your feet turn in or out? What part of your foot hits the floor first? The toes? The outer edge? The heel? Are your feet landing toes in (pigeon toe) or toes out (slew foot)?

Be aware of what your knees are doing. Does the knee snap back tightly into a locked position at the end of each step, and does it begin the next stiffly? Do you roll up onto your toes at each step or shuffle your feet? What happens at your hips? Do you swing them side to side? Is one side stiffer?

What is your torso doing? Do you feel any tension in the small of your back? Do you keep your torso upright as you move forward, or do you lean over?

What does your head do at each step? Perhaps it bobs up and down or leads your body.

Write down these observations about the way you walk.

Locking the knees and pitching the pelvis too far forward are indications of basic misalignment.

SITTING

Right off the bat, I must tell you that it is practically impossible to sit both correctly and comfortably in a chair. Most chairs are so constructed that maintaining correct alignment while sitting in them is out of the question. They're the wrong size, the wrong shape, and the wrong degree of firmness.

Sit down in any chair and take note of the following points: Can the small of your back press up against the back of the chair? If it's an upholstered armchair, the answer is probably no. Can your feet rest flat on the floor? The seats of many chairs are too long from front to back for anyone under five foot four inches or so. You have to slide forward in the seat if your feet are to reach the floor, so that you must correspondingly slouch, resting the middle of your back against the back of the chair— you cannot sit straight in it.

And what's happening to your neck as you sit slouched back in this soft chair that is probably not giving you any support? Is it retracted, pulled in on itself, or does it arch forward so that you can balance your head only with effort? Is it straining to find balance in an unbalanced position?

Think of your body as a whole. How compressed is your upper body when you sit in a chair? Do your legs drop outward or inward, causing knee strain? As the small of your back collapses, seeking support, it puts a strain on the lower back, which is now stretched out in a position of stress that is the opposite of swayback. The shoulders, too, are likely (since there is no support from the lower back) to round forward, hunching over and collapsing the chest and creating tension in the neck.

The situation is even worse when it comes to car seats. If you're over five foot four, you have to crank your seat back almost flat to give your legs room enough to stretch out. In cars and trucks that have no variable seat back adjustment, it's worse yet: the small of your back gets no support at all. You are constantly thrown too far behind the line of gravity, which would normally run from the top of the head down through the shoulder and hip. Anytime you're out of its flow, gravity presses you down, causing pain.

Some of these problems can be prevented. Use chairs that are not too high. Make sure that your legs form a right angle to the floor and that your back forms a right angle with the seat. Place as many pillows as you need behind your back so that you can relax a little and still be held upright.

Two cases of bad posture.

Slouching in a sitting position puts strain on the lower back and creates tension in the neck.

TAKING THE STANCE

Now we'll address each part of your body as you learn the Stance. You will become aware of how and where you feel strange when you're lined up on the grid of the Stance. Know that you *will* feel very different; your old way was comfortable, habitual, yet we've seen that it was responsible for pain and debility.

The key to Balanced Alignment is, first, an accurate

The stranger the new way feels, the better.

sense of what you're doing, what it feels like as well as what it looks like, and any difference between the two. As you go through the Stance in front of a mirror, you'll learn from visual feedback that what you now know is correct, symmetrical and balanced will *look* good but will *feel* very awkward, stiff and impossible to maintain. If, for instance, you've been habitually

holding one shoulder higher than the other for some time, chances are this unevenness felt "straight"—when in fact one shoulder is visibly higher than the other and you may even be tilting your whole upper body over to one side. Now that you *know* you should be level, tension occurs because the new way, the Stance, feels so different and awkward. *This discrepancy is what we are trying to create.* This is where change will take place. This feeling is what signals the brain to decide to let the body actually change the programing rather than simply to try something new, then revert back to the old way. By placing yourself in the Stance, and maintaining it with your breath, coupled with doing the movements in the next chapter to loosen your body enough to accept the change, you specifically lengthen and strengthen the precise muscles that have been pulling you awry. This is the only effective way to change your lifelong habits, which is our ultimate goal. Then this new way will in turn become

Proper alignment of the foot allows the arch to lift and form a supportive "bridge" as part of the Stance foundation.

habitual, so that staying with it will not depend on "will power."

A precise awareness of such discrepancies is essential before you can change. You must see what you're doing and feel it *accurately* so that ultimately you'll be able to sense it without having to look.

● **ELASTIC BAND**
The foundation of the Stance starts with the feet hip-width apart and pointing *straight ahead,* with the weight of the feet centered along a straight line from the base of the second toe to the center of the heel. At right angles to this line is the horizontal line of the ankle bones.

As you align your feet and ankles, feel what it now becomes

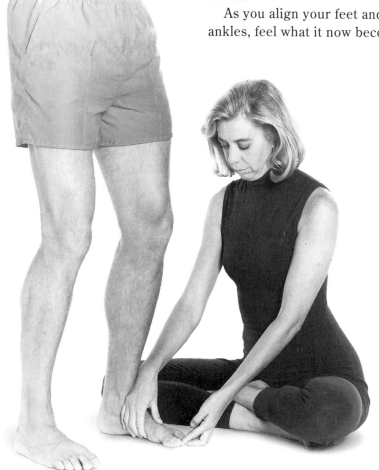

STRENGTH THROUGH FLEXIBILITY

SCOTT'S STORY

Scott, a young figure skater from New York, came to my group classes in Sun Valley one summer because he'd been having trouble landing his triple axels (a complicated maneuver that involves jumping, turning three times in the air and landing on one skate) and his coach thought he would benefit from some alignment work.

We were all surprised and appalled when he tried to do the Ankle Sit: not only was he unable to sit back flat on his ankles, but he couldn't even begin to fold his feet underneath him! His feet were frozen—fixed at a right angle—just as if he were still wearing skates. It was amazing that he could skate at all, let alone as well as he did, considering the extent of his handicap.

As the summer progressed, Scott began slowly to make headway in releasing and opening his ankles. Starting with a large pile of pillows beneath his buttocks, he progressed bit by bit until he was at last able to fold his feet underneath him and rest back on the pillows. Then began the work of stretching and opening the front of his feet and shins. This was very slow and difficult; he had skated several hours a day for fifteen years, always with rigidly fixed

ankles. It took an entire summer, working four hours a week, for him finally to relax enough to sit back on his ankles without the pillows.

Along with the restoration of flexibility came a new strength and power: stretching the muscles of his feet and shins allowed his Achilles tendon to contract enough to be able to lengthen. For the first time in his skating career, he was able to bend at the ankles and thus bend enough at the knees to get the spring for a higher jump. This extra lift gave him the ease to turn properly in the air and land squarely over his skate. It was this new flexibility in his lower legs that made available to him greater strength in his quadriceps muscles (the front of the thighs).

Scott was astonished by two things: how tight he'd been, and how loose he'd become. "It's quite a paradox that as I become less rigid in my ankles, I'm getting *stronger*," he said. "I'd always thought strength *was* tightness— an unmoving fixed grip. Now I see it's just the reverse. The deeper I can flex my joints, the more time I have on my spins; I'm not constantly almost late. Also, I can now land my jumps with reliable accuracy—not the hit-or-miss chanciness of before."

possible to do with the "bridge" of your arch. Notice how you're able to engage the complex and subtle foot and leg muscles so that they can lift from within to create an arch. As you do the Thirty-Four Movements in the next chapter, you'll find that the muscles of your feet will soon become more flexible and much stronger, giving you a far more reliable base of support.

Now think of maintaining the tension on the imaginary ELASTIC BAND as you roll your ankles outward to lift your arches. Become aware of how different from your old way of standing this may feel, especially if you have flat feet and your foot muscles are weak. Be willing to stay with, and become familiar with, this strange new feeling.

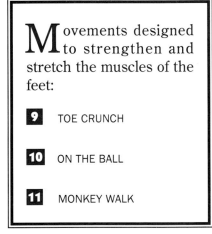

Movements designed to strengthen and stretch the muscles of the feet:

9 TOE CRUNCH

10 ON THE BALL

11 MONKEY WALK

- **FELT-TIPPED MARKERS**

Notice also where your ankles must be for the FELT-TIPPED MARKERS to be aimed so that they are parallel to the floor. If you corrected by rolling your ankles too far outward, make them

---

The ankle joint lays the foundation for everything that happens above it.

---

parallel by rolling them a little to the inside; if they are rolled too far inward, roll them a little to the outside. When you consciously apply this rotational pressure, either outward or inward, making small but definite shifts in weight distribution, you begin to engage very subtle muscles throughout the entire foot, leg and hip.

Your ankle joints are probably not as open and flexible as they can be; most of us move on stiff, unbending ankle joints. If the ankles are not fully mobile, the knees cannot move freely, nor can the hips. This prevents

the spine from moving to the correct placement over the feet so that it can move correctly with gravity. Thus we see that stiff or "frozen" ankle joints pass on their immobility all the way up the body, reducing range of motion and inducing stiffness everywhere.

Movements that are especially helpful in opening the ankle joints and lower legs:

5 HEEL DROP ON STAIRS

12 SQUAT AND REACH

15 STAIR CLIMB, UP AND DOWN

16 GROUCHO WALK

18 ANKLE SIT

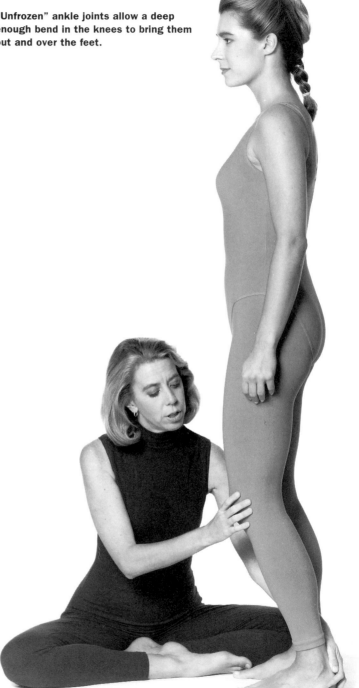

"Unfrozen" ankle joints allow a deep enough bend in the knees to bring them out and over the feet.

• **HEADLIGHTS**

Where are your kneecaps facing? Do your HEADLIGHTS shine straight ahead or do they angle off to the side?

What correction must you make to have your knees point straight ahead? Are they in line with your second toes? If you have to make an adjustment to line up your HEADLIGHTS, watch the effect this adjustment has on the small of your back and the tops of your buttocks. If you have knock-knees, in particular, you'll need to learn how to move your legs farther apart at the knees so that they line up straight. Feel what bringing your HEADLIGHTS into line does to the small of your back—can you sense how it opens up the congestion in this area?

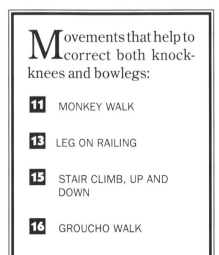

Movements that help to correct both knock-knees and bowlegs:

11 MONKEY WALK

13 LEG ON RAILING

15 STAIR CLIMB, UP AND DOWN

16 GROUCHO WALK

• **HARPOONS**

Now, with your feet and ankles in the Stance and your HEADLIGHTS pointing straight ahead, think of HARPOONS dangling from your kneecaps. Do the tips aim straight down toward the tops of your feet? To bring them out and over your feet, to a point just ahead of the second toe, you must *bend your knees*. Feel how aligning your knees, ankles and feet immediately takes pressure off your back.

People with knee pain usually are not hinging the leg with the knee over the foot and in line with the second toe. You will probably have to correct by leaning farther forward from your ankles and bending your knees more deeply to get the tips of the knees in line with the edge of the toes. If you do, be sure to keep your heels firmly planted on the floor as well. (Your weight is still centered, not rocked back on your heels. The point here is simply not to let your heels rise off the ground.) This two-way press, firmly down with the weight of the feet *and* down through the thighs, will help you to balance as you drive the tips of the HARPOONS into the floor.

THE POWER OF THE STANCE

ELLEN'S STORY

Ellen, a waitress in her mid-thirties, came to me with chronic lower back pain. She couldn't afford many lessons, so we decided to see how far we could get in just one session. Apart from her discomfort she was in very good shape, strong and limber, and had no other complaints.

As I always do, I started by taking her through the Stance. As soon as we reached the knees and hips, she realized at once what was causing her back pain. She was creating it herself by locking her knees; this in turn gave her a swayback, which led her to thrust a hip out to one side in order to relieve the tension from the locked knees and swayback. She stayed in this position for hours at a stretch, since she was on her feet so much, and her lower back was rebelling against the continuous stress.

The pain disappeared completely once she understood—and felt, as we progressed through the Stance—that her torso could lift *upward*, buoyed by the energy sent *down from her hips*, through her legs, to her feet. In this way, pressure was not forcing her hip out to the side, causing her pain. Not only could she now stay on her feet without discomfort, but she also experienced new energy and power from the unlocking of blocked knee and hip joints.

• RACCOON EYES

The hinges where your thighs meet your hips are the points where the RACCOON EYES peer out—sleepily when the hinges are partially closed, wide open when the hinges are open.

What can you do to widen the angle between your hip joints and torso so that the RACCOON EYES open wide? You must squeeze your buttocks slightly, in effect rotating your thighs around to the back and keeping your legs firm there, securing them in this back position. Be sure your knees (and ankles) are well hinged as you tighten these muscles. Later, after your hips and ankles open sufficiently, you won't have to squeeze your buttocks to keep the hinge open and your thighs rotated around to the back.

Opening the angle between the tops of your thighs and your torso lengthens your lower back and allows your upper body to rise straight up from your pelvis. As you experience this new sensation of length and height, keep in mind that increasing the space between your joints to lengthen your body is one of the most important changes we'll accomplish in the Stance.

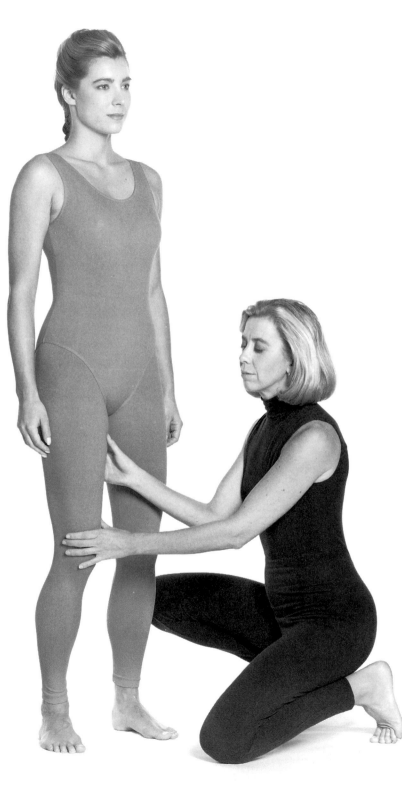

The letter "H." Now check to see that your hip joints are in the position to form the tops of the letter "H," with your legs as the two outer straight lines and your knees as the crosspieces.

Feel what you're doing in your thighs and ankles to separate one leg from the other enough to form the "H." This external pressure, if you have knock-knees, is important for releasing your hip joints and may well feel as if you're being asked to stand like a cowboy, with room enough for a horse between your legs. If you have bowlegs, the challenge will be to bring your legs more to center and square with the feet. It is essential for Balanced Alignment that your legs be directly under your pelvis, not curved out.

Squeezing the buttocks slightly rotates the thighs around to the back, separating one leg from the other to form the end pieces of the letter "H."

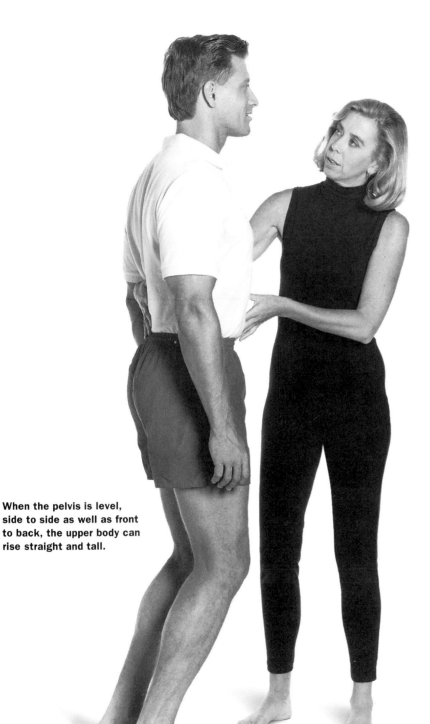

When the pelvis is level, side to side as well as front to back, the upper body can rise straight and tall.

● PAIL OF WATER

At the top of your hips is the rim of the PAIL OF WATER that represents your pelvis and buttocks. To make the rim level, so that the water doesn't spill out the front or back, pull in your abdomen. As you tighten the muscles in this area, the small of your back will also flatten to help keep the pail level. Again, this is a temporary, artificial gripping that will not be needed later on.

Feel the connection between your abdomen and back as the muscles in these areas work together to support your spinal column. At the same time, think of lengthening your torso between your hips and your waist.

Remember, our goal is *length, length, and more length.*

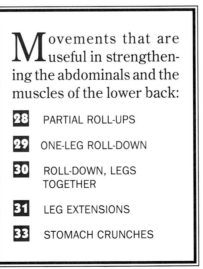

Movements that are useful in strengthening the abdominals and the muscles of the lower back:

28	PARTIAL ROLL-UPS
29	ONE-LEG ROLL-DOWN
30	ROLL-DOWN, LEGS TOGETHER
31	LEG EXTENSIONS
33	STOMACH CRUNCHES

STANCE CHECK

We have now come halfway through the Stance. Let's return to your old way of standing for a moment to see how different it feels. Allow your legs to revert to their usual position. Look what's happened to your feet: turned out? Your knees: locked? Your pelvis: tilted back? Your legs: angled in? Feel whether any of your old, habitual pain creeps in and sense that this pain is caused by how you are standing and holding yourself in space. Begin to be aware that there is more than one "setting" for your body, that you have now experienced two of them, and that you know what the difference between them feels like.

We are aiming at an alignment in which the feet are straight ahead, the knees straight ahead and bent quite a bit (at first you may have to bend them more sharply, more than you think you should, until your leg muscles have lengthened and your hip joints have become free), the torso rising straight up out of the hips, which have opened up to allow this, and the PAIL OF WATER perfectly level from front to back. Note that in reverting to your old standing position, your feet may have moved apart because your ankles, rolling back in again, may have taken a wider stance in order for you to try to keep your balance. This gives your lower half an "A" shape, like the outline of an A-frame house, with the narrowest part at the top and the widest at the bottom. If this looks awkward to you, you may already be beginning to sense that there is something wrong about the way you hold your body.

Now return to the Stance, placing your feet, ankles, knees and hips in our new alignment. Notice how the proper bending at the ankles and knees tends to release the lower back into length, reducing the compression of the spine, lengthening the natural curve there (at the lumbar spine) and thus eliminating the swayback that most people have at least to some degree. Since the swayback is no longer pushing the belly forward, it has room to drop back. However, even with maximum bending of the ankles and knees, the abdominal muscles may be so weak that they still pull the lower back forward and your belly still sags.

We want to train the spine to be sturdy and upright, through the coordinated effort of the abdominal and back muscles.

Feel how opening the RACCOON EYES is helping to keep the PAIL OF WATER level, and vice versa. Each correction enhances the other. The health of the spine depends on the lower spine being released, free of compression. We achieve this stretching first by flattening the small of the back, strengthening and engaging the abdominal muscles, then lengthening the muscles of the back; front and back together give a firm girdle of support for the spine.

Next, we want to lift your entire torso up and out of your hips. Sometimes the tendency is to correct the swayback by tucking the pelvis under but then failing to lift the upper body out of the lower so that the spine curves and compresses. It is with our next image that you will trigger your mind actually to lift the upper body up and away from the waist.

Remember, *it is what we do below the hips that determines the ease and balance above them.*

RED HERRINGS

LOUISE'S STORY

What was particularly interesting about Louise's case was the way we got to the source of her problem. Louise, an attractive woman in her fifties, had pulled a hamstring in her left leg in a fall. Now she complained of an immobilizing pain in her left hip. We went through the Stance together and saw that she had hammertoes, bunions and knock-knees (all of them more severe on the left side). She also had a little potbelly.

As we worked on releasing and strengthening the hamstring, she began to experience the sensation of the connection between her foot and her knee, and her knee to her hip. Releasing the hip joint helped the pain in her hip. But when we began to work on strengthening her buttocks so that she could hold her left leg in correct alignment, we discovered that she had next to no strength or control on the entire outer side of her left leg. It had taken the impact of the fall, and she had almost lost feeling there because of a pinched nerve.

We would never have found the real trouble if we hadn't methodically released her enough to reach that vulnerable spot. Even her potbelly yielded when we corrected her alignment. With both legs straight and facing directly ahead, she could hold her pelvis more easily upright, allowing her abdominal and back muscles to work in tandem and her stomach to flatten dramatically.

"My parents both became decrepit at a pretty young age," said Louise, "and I just thought it was my turn. I certainly never imagined that working on the pain in my hip would help to straighten my crooked toes and knees—they'd been that way ever since I could remember. All those old aches and pains are gone now, too. It really *is* all connected, isn't it? I'd never have believed it—I feel good now for another fifty thousand miles!"

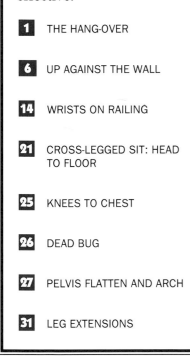

Many of the Thirty-Four Movements are useful in lengthening the spine. The following movements are particularly effective:

1 THE HANG-OVER

6 UP AGAINST THE WALL

14 WRISTS ON RAILING

21 CROSS-LEGGED SIT: HEAD TO FLOOR

25 KNEES TO CHEST

26 DEAD BUG

27 PELVIS FLATTEN AND ARCH

31 LEG EXTENSIONS

- **SHIMS**

How will you create the inner space between your ribs and hips to make room for the SHIMS that lengthen your torso? Do you feel like locking your knees to stabilize yourself for *more length*?

Resist the temptation to lock; keep your knees bent and forward, and allow the length to come from the two-way flow of energy—of gravity *flowing down* from the waist and of the energy stream *rising* from the waist. The torso will not get the message that it is safe enough to really *lift* until the heels are securely planted. It is the pressing down, through feet and legs that can accept the pressure, that tells the torso to lift. So it is not that you are relying on will power; the lifting comes as a natural result of pressing down! This lift and flow from the waist allows you to separate your upper torso from your lower torso and gives you a narrow, elegant waistline.

Pressing down on the heels allows the torso to lift, buoyed by the stream of energy rising from the waist.

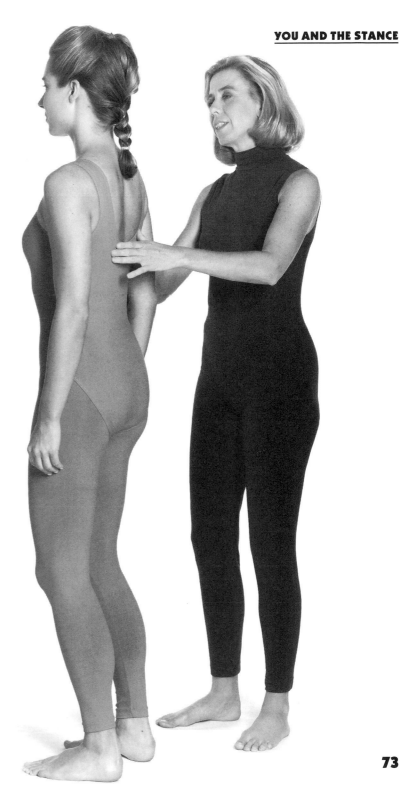

• PLUNGER

The chest area (around the breastbone, or sternum) should be easily tall and flat, not hunched over. What must you do to keep the handle of the PLUNGER sticking out from your chest parallel to the ground? What must you do with *your whole body* to keep the handle from drooping toward the ground? You must *lengthen your torso*. Feel how tall you are now in the midriff (between navel and breastbone), and yet how well grounded by the flow of gravity moving down through your legs. You will have a new sense of spaciousness opening up in your lower back.

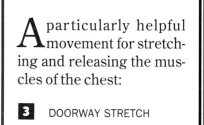

A particularly helpful movement for stretching and releasing the muscles of the chest:

3 DOORWAY STRETCH

4 ARMS BEHIND ON RAILING

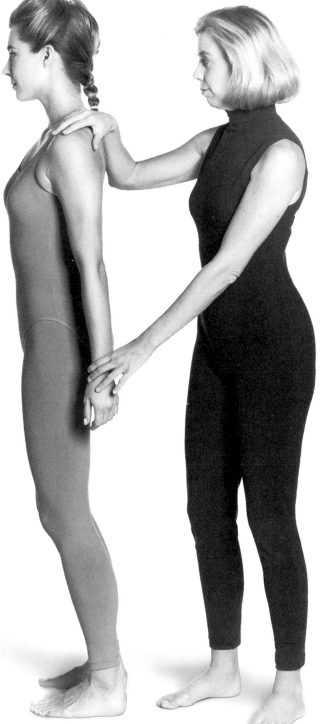

• MILKMAID'S YOKE

Look at the position of your shoulders. Is the MILKMAID'S YOKE perfectly level, parallel to the ground? What must you do to make your shoulders straight across, not raised or curved? You must press them back and down, *contracting* between the shoulder blades and *stretching* across the front of the chest. Holding one or both shoulders high and pulled into the neck tends to shorten and tighten the muscles of the upper back and neck—and even those of the back of the head.

Moreover, since they are not suspended from any structural support, the shoulders often pull forward if they are not correctly aligned. These rounded shoulders press the whole chest downward and inward, collapsing it with a heavy downward pressure and creating tension in the neck.

In proper alignment, the shoulders are carried back and down, opening the chest and strengthening the upper back.

Opening the shoulders, freeing them to widen out to either side, tends to release this entire group of muscles—those of the upper back and neck—as well as the muscles down the arms.

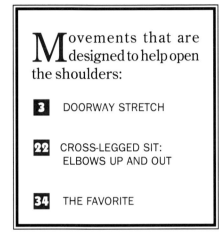

Movements that are designed to help open the shoulders:

3 DOORWAY STRETCH

22 CROSS-LEGGED SIT: ELBOWS UP AND OUT

34 THE FAVORITE

REGAINING MOBILITY

SETH'S STORY

Seth, a man in his sixties, came to me with an exaggerated case of one of the most common problems in my older clients: a loss of mobility in the upper back that curves it forward and slumps it down. His back had been sharply curved and hunched for many years due to a sailing accident in his youth. The pain from this extreme stoop had at last become so severe that he could no longer even play golf. In addition, because of his "hump" (the upper spinal curve amounted to that), he couldn't wear his expensive new suit.

He often despaired of ever changing and remained dissatisfied no matter how many breakthroughs he achieved—for example, being able finally to do the Ankle Sit with no pillows underneath his thighs after needing four to start with, or when he could straighten both legs while keeping his hands flat on the floor. He wanted to stand tall again, with no "hump" in his back. Nothing else would do.

To gain access to his back, we first lengthened his hamstrings. All the muscles of the front of his torso were short and tight, and the opposing muscles of his back were weak and overstretched, so we worked first on opening and

releasing the muscles of his chest and next on strengthening the muscles in his back so that they could support him upright. In effect, we had to uncurl him, as though his whole upper body were a curled-up postage stamp that needed to be flattened out. When the supporting muscles were long enough, his spine lengthened amazingly. Of course, the spine is an extraordinarily flexible column—as is obvious when you consider the seemingly infinite variety of ways it can become twisted and distorted—so the improvement can be equally startling.

Seth's moment of victory came when he put on his new suit and took part in his church's Easter service. Tall, straight and confident, he carried the wine down the aisle to the applause of the entire congregation. All his determination and hard work paid off in that one proud moment.

Seth says, "It sure feels different, standing straight again. The pain in my lower back is gone—and it used to wake me up every night, it was so bad. The other pain, between my shoulder blades, only comes back when I slouch. And now I can look in the mirror and see myself as I was all those years ago, before my accident."

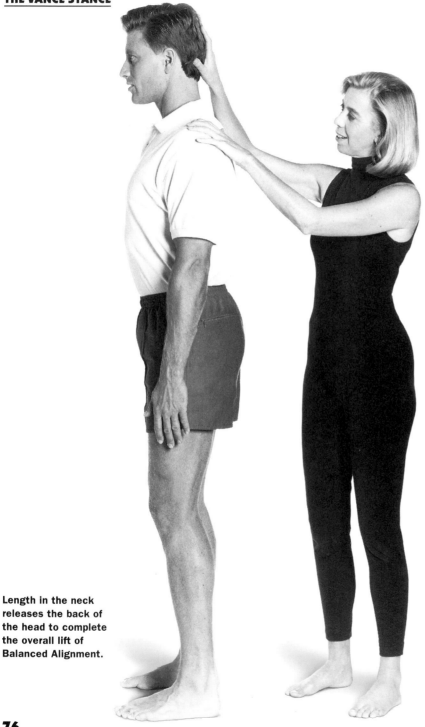

Length in the neck releases the back of the head to complete the overall lift of Balanced Alignment.

● ACCORDION

Where is your neck? What must your neck do to be balanced easily under your head? Yes— it must *lengthen*. As you become more centered over your feet, your neck moves forward in space, aligned for lifting. Feel how light and effortless it is when your body below the neck is in Balanced Alignment. Feel what you must do to stretch out this imaginary ACCORDION along a vertical line. Notice how little correction is needed in the proper horizontal line of your chin to feel quite clearly the one place that is the most comfortable. You are beginning to be able to tune in to how sensitive your body is.

The neck is both delicate and strong, a miracle of design. When traveling in South America, I marveled at the way men carried all manner of objects from straps wrapped around their foreheads and hanging down their backs, with the weight borne principally by the neck. Firewood, furniture, even heavy machinery were all transported by "neck power." Women, too, carried enormous bundles of washing and buckets of water on their head, again using only neck power. These people all seemed to know the secret that *correct alignment gives power to the body* and that our sense of having weak necks comes from letting them sink down into our chests or holding them out unnaturally.

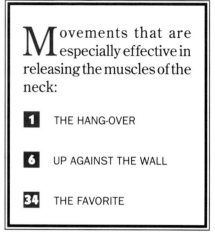

Movements that are especially effective in releasing the muscles of the neck:

1 THE HANG-OVER

6 UP AGAINST THE WALL

34 THE FAVORITE

● GOLDEN HOOK

As your neck lengthens, feel what you must do to attach the GOLDEN HOOK to the imaginary "eye" above.

You have just connected the upper part of your spine to the back of your neck. Now you are releasing the back of your head to rise up from inside your neck. Once your spine, topped off by your head, is lifted as long as it was designed to be, your entire body is participating as a unified, integrated whole in this business of standing.

● **PIECE OF PAPER**

Now, as your body reaches up to attach the GOLDEN HOOK, remember what helps you stay firmly planted: your PIECE OF PAPER. Feel how you *stretch* the backs of your legs to press down and how the shins *contract*. This supplies the pressure that keeps the PIECE OF PAPER under your heels.

Feel also how this helps the SHIMS between your ribs to keep separating and lengthening, and the PLUNGER extending from your chest to stay straight and parallel to the ground.

When you are properly aligned from foot to head, the middle of your foot and the midpoint of your hips (as seen from the side) are in a straight line. As the RACCOON EYES are opened wide, your weight is shifted ever so slightly forward from the hips up through the top of your head. That is, the opening of the RACCOON EYES sends your upper body out in space, no longer settled back on your heels (which we never want) but centered over your feet. This, together with your knees being quite bent, produces a feeling of being angled slightly forward.

You may need to bend your knees quite sharply for a while, until the muscles along the outsides of your legs have lengthened somewhat and your ankles have become more flexible. Eventually you won't need such a sharp bend in the knees and can just keep them lightly and easily flexed.

THE ENERGY STREAM

With your body *more forward* and *more lifted,* you will experience the feeling of being carried upward on the energy stream. Confusion often arises over the word "forward." Should you actually *lean* or *bend* forward, as if washing at a low sink? Absolutely not. "Forward" refers to the placement of your entire body, starting at your feet and ankles and projecting in a line up through the top of your head.

It is a line that bisects the foot, right in the center of the arch, then rises through the middle of the knee, in its more deeply bent position. It then travels up through the pelvis, straight up through the torso at the level of the shoulders, through the center of the neck, and bisects the head at the ear.

Again, this *magical line of power and strength* begins at a point farther forward on the foot than most of us are accustomed to. The unifying concept of a tall tree, with directional energies running both up and down, sap running up the trunk and roots growing down into the earth, is useful here. Both directional energies are essential if the tree is to grow tall and strong. The sap lifts the trunk up and the roots grow far down into the earth, anchoring the tree so that it can extend upward without falling over or pulling the roots out. So too with the body. It needs both anchoring and uplifting to be able to exist in gravity with no effort.

Contrast this way of standing with your old way, in which the energy—or sap, in our tree image—was *pooling downward.* When you tried to stand up "straight," your effort *pushed* the energy *upward,* artificially, as in a toothpaste tube being squeezed. You could never keep yourself erect because this was *effortful* posture. When you tried to stand up taller with your knees locked, your knees could not act independently of your torso. Any impulse you sent to your spine was waylaid by the locked joints. And so, although you believed you were asking your body to stand up tall and straight, you were actually reinforcing and exaggerating what you were already doing. You did the same thing in childhood, when to be taller meant to do *more* of what you did in the first place to become upright and mobile—which was to lock your knees.

Existing effortlessly in gravity depends on pressing down with your feet as you lift from your waist.

In the Stance, you will break the habit of trying to become taller by locking your knees. To repeat: *Never again lock your knees!* You will also learn to keep your PAIL OF WATER level and your spine erect, so that it will be the *spine* that responds when you give yourself the command to lift, neither your knees nor your pelvis pushing upward. And since you will be angled slightly "forward," it will be easier to maintain this uprightness because you'll be in the energy stream, the line of gravity on which its negative effects are nullified. You will actually be taller, even with your knees bent!

Now, instead of having to choose between being set back on your heels or pitched forward, on the brink of falling on your face, you have a third option: *to be balanced on your feet,* with your weight distributed evenly from heel to toe. Here you are neither just lifting up nor settled back and down. Rather, by being slightly angled "forward," you are asking energy to flow up and down at once. To maintain this forward angling, however, you must do something to keep your heels from rising up off the ground. If you're not anchored at your feet, your spine cannot be free to stretch out to its full length. It is by affixing your feet that you can lean that much farther forward, and lift that much taller, than before. Pressing down on the PIECE OF PAPER while lifting up to attach the GOLDEN HOOK is what allows you to send the energy *in both directions.* (Lead ski boots on a magnetic floor would also do the trick!)

This pressure in your heels as you come upright and lift *releases* very subtle pressure in your neck, allowing your head to float up. You are beginning to stand in Balanced Alignment, using its power to lift you up and anchor

Only when your body is in Balanced Alignment, each part working in harmony with every other part, can you experience the power, lightness and ease intended by nature.

you firmly. Only in this relationship with gravity are you an integral whole, every part working harmoniously with every other part. Only now are you safe from deceptive compensations in which you unconsciously choose the expedient over the powerful, the short-term convenience over long-term health and efficiency. And only here will you experience the lightness, ease and joy of your body at its optimum "setting," free from unbalanced drag.

At this precise placement is where the body works best, with the least effort and strain. There are many other possible settings that work pretty well—for a while. But for the long haul (and that means anytime past the age of thirty) you must constantly seek that point of Balanced Alignment, that line of power on the energy stream.

Now that you have the Stance as a model, you can think your

way up your body from feet to head, establishing the relationship between the body parts—joints and straight pieces—in the new, released Balanced Alignment (ankles well flexed, knees flexed over the feet, hips open, waistline level, and so on all the way up) that places you precisely on the energy stream in the position of maximum easy lift. Instead of a continual struggle against a downward drag, standing will be an experience of flowing power.

FEELING LIKE FRANKENSTEIN?

At this point, having worked your way through the Stance with an awareness of your own particular problems and obstacles, you may feel that you could never make this way of standing feel natural, let alone flowing and relaxed. You may feel more like a lurching monster, unnaturally

stiff and awkward. You may even find that you're holding your breath.

Don't worry. The thing to remember is that *the stranger it feels at first, the better.* We must become aware of our problems, recognize that they are *specific* problems, and identify them more and more precisely, locate them, and trace them to their source. All this is part of the developing awareness that must become second nature before the Balanced Alignment of the Stance can do so.

If you're feeling strange, it's because muscles that have been inactive or were never used are slowly coming to life. For now, just let yourself *feel* how different the new way is from your old way, without judgment. Let yourself be the beginner on the new path of awareness. I can guarantee you that the Stance will become increasingly more comfortable, feel more natural, as you repeatedly go through it, releasing tight muscles, freeing stiff joints by a deliberate act of awareness that focuses your attention on each part of your body systematically, from feet to head.

In the next chapter, we'll go through the Thirty-Four Movements that will stretch and strengthen the muscles that need to be reactivated, bringing them back into play as they assume new roles in Balanced Alignment. If you practice the movements regularly, you'll find that running through the Stance becomes increasingly easy and that it becomes (and this is the real promise of the Stance) *integrated into everything you do, a part of every aspect of your life.*

You'll be newly aware of all the ways you use your body that you previously took for granted, in the simplest actions, such as standing and walking and sitting. You'll decide whether or not you're performing these actions the way you want to perform them, the way you were designed to perform them, the ideal way, or simply making do in a way that is inefficient, damaging and painful, and limits your possibilities.

NOW YOU HAVE A CHOICE

Working through the Stance and looking closely at your particular habits and problems, at where you personally are right now in relation to the ideal of Balanced Alignment, you begin to acquire a choice in how you use yourself—for better or for worse. What we have done together in this chapter is the first step in changing from habit to awareness, and the choice you now have is clear. You can continue operating in your old unthinking, habitual mode, or you can change to the mode of conscious awareness. You can continue unthinkingly, using your body as an interlocking system of locked joints and increasing the damage and deterioration day by day, or you can change through becoming conscious of what you're doing and replacing it with a balanced relationship of muscles and joints that will reverse past damage and prevent damage in the future—as well as giving you a new pleasure in using your body in the here and now.

If you wanted to, you'd probably be able to drive your car improperly and still manage to get to your destination—at the cost of completely unnecessary and excessive wear and tear. For example, you *could* drive with one foot riding the brake pedal while holding the other down on the gas pedal, wearing out the brakes and straining the engine. And you *could* drive with poorly aligned tires and not even know you were wearing down the tread prematurely. But most of us don't need to be told not to do these things—we understand automatically that a properly maintained car functions better and lasts longer.

With awareness comes responsibility for your own well-being.

For some reason, however, we tend not to extend this concept to the machine that is our body, until it sends us unmistakable signals that we can no longer ignore. Most of my clients have come to me simply because they were in trouble and had heard that I might be able to help them. The fact that my help consisted not in passive manipulation, massage or something they could "take" to make them feel better, but rather in engaging their deep sense of intuition that *this* part of the body affected *that* part and that the vague feeling of not being "quite right" had a specific source, came as a surprise. But the extent of their improvement, and the vastly expanded potential for removing the causes of most pain when they learned the simple techniques of the Vance Stance program, came as an even bigger surprise.

In this chapter, we've begun the first part of the program: developing an awareness of how you have been most of your life and becoming acquainted with a new ideal of alignment, the Stance. In the next chapter, you'll learn the Thirty-Four Movements that will enable you to transform your body so that it becomes one with this new ideal. By doing these movements, you will make the Stance part of your daily reality.

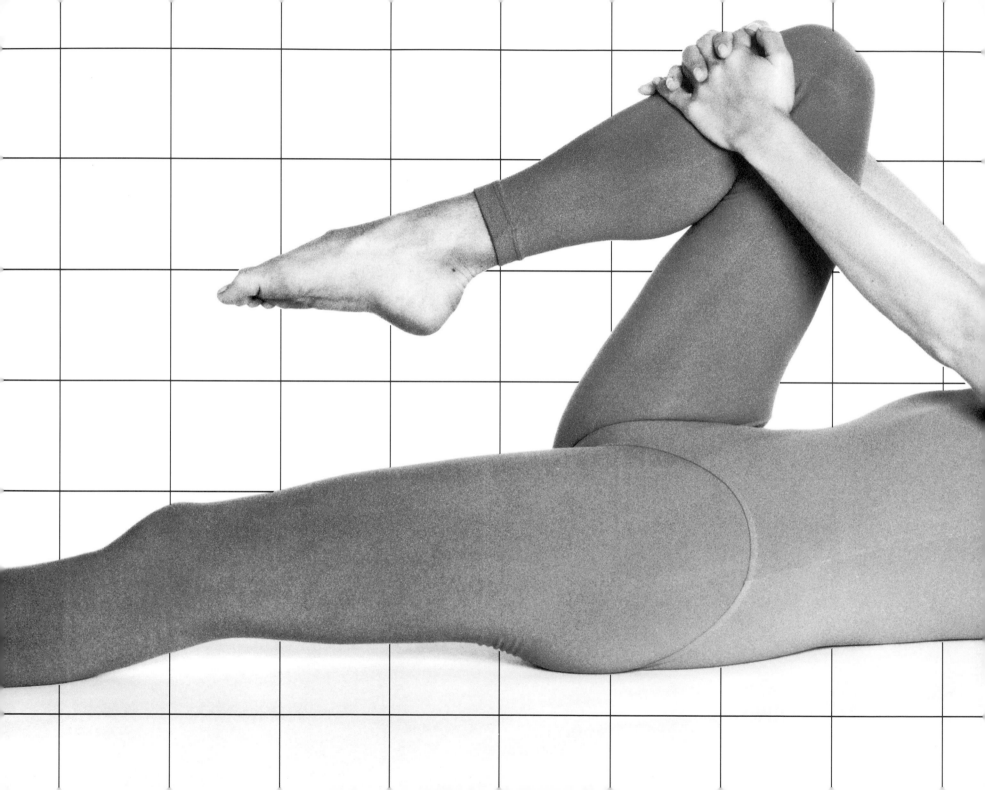

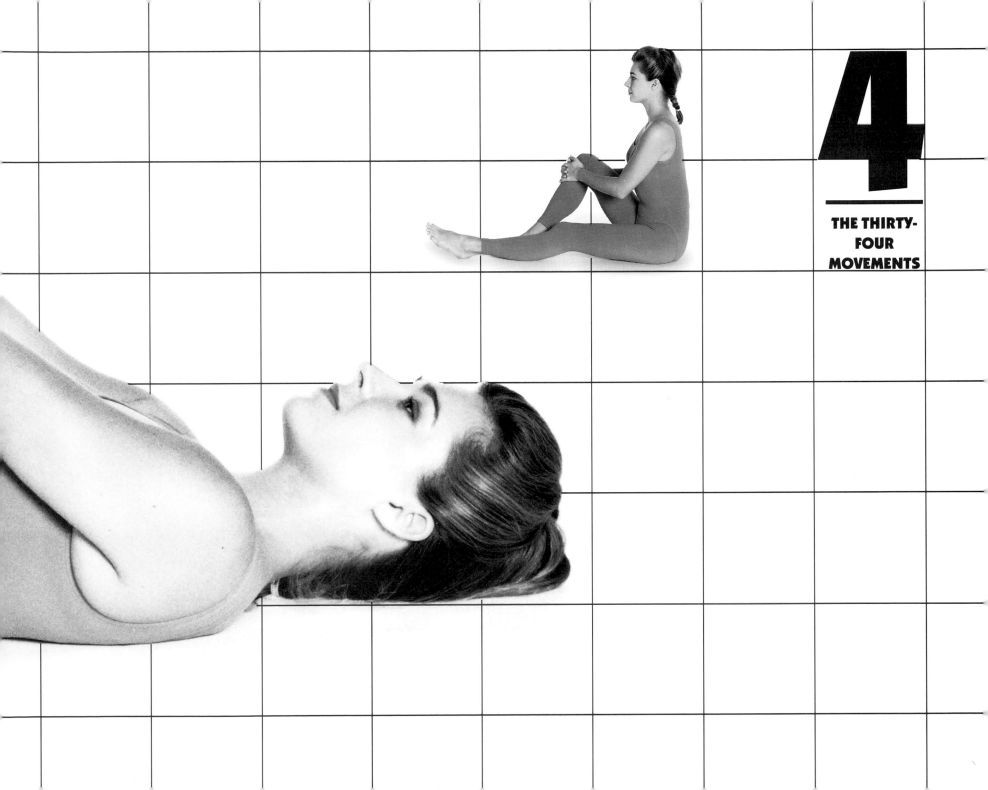

4

THE THIRTY-
FOUR
MOVEMENTS

CHAPTER FOUR

THE THIRTY-FOUR MOVE-MENTS

By now you should be thoroughly familiar with the Stance, at least as an ideal—a goal that, when reached, will put you in perfect Balanced Alignment. You know what it is; now you'll learn how to get there.

The Thirty-Four Movements that follow are intended to make it possible for you to *live* in the Balanced Alignment of the Stance. Each of them stretches and strengthens muscle groups that need to be activated before the Stance can become second nature.

FLEXIBILITY, THEN STRENGTH

The emphasis here is on flexibility, because muscles that are elastic and flexible—that can lengthen and compress— are also strong. As explained in Chapter Two, there are two ways in which muscles can be inadequate to their job of holding you up and moving you around. They can be overstretched or slack, or they can be too tight and contracted; either way, they are weak. In other words, muscles can be too long or too short—as a permanent condition.

Ideally, muscles should be as *elastic* as possible, capable of both contracting fully and lengthening fully. It is the loss of flexibility that most interferes with your ability to assume and maintain the easy efficiency of the Stance, and so it is on flexibility that the Thirty-Four Movements are focused. Strength will follow as all the areas that have been blocked to strength are opened and we do some more specific movements to build your strength gradually. As you become increasingly straighter in limbs and torso, and your joints and muscles become more limber, you will notice strength without having done much that appears strengthening.

Through our work together, you are bringing into play muscles that you may have never known you had. As you repeat the movements, you'll find it easier and easier to call on these newly awakened muscles as they enter more fully into your awareness and become stronger and stronger. Make a point of concentrating on these muscles, however weak and unwilling they seem at first. If you cultivate them, they will rapidly increase in strength.

THE "S" SOUND

Breathing is the mechanism that effects change in the body. When you ask your body to do something different from what it's been doing in the past, your brain needs a clear signal to proceed. It needs to know that this change is a desirable one despite the body's resistance. Breathing as *if* you were already comfortable in a new position overrides pain's negative message to stop with a message of assurance: "I must be okay, because I'm breathing in a relaxed full manner." The body then lets go of the tightness to make the message be true.

What is not always understood is that the tightness tends to occur not so much on the *inhale* as on the *exhale*. (If you exhale properly, the inhale will take care of itself.) An easy way to focus on the exhale is to make an "S" sound, like a hiss, as in "s-s-s-s- snake." This way you hear the exhale continuing throughout the movement, and you have better control than you would with the "whoosh" release that comes from blowing the breath out through an open mouth.

Be aware that, as you

STRETCHING AS RELEASING

Stretching is often thought to be a pulling to get the muscles to lengthen, like pulling down a too-short T-shirt. More correctly, it is asking and allowing the muscle to let go, to release from within, like relaxing your arm after carrying a heavy suitcase.

Locked parts of the body are very sensitive, and releasing them needs to be approached gently, nothing abrupt or violent, so that you feel safe as you go along in the stretch; otherwise, the body/mind is likely to react by clamping down even tighter than before. As you become aware of tightness and stiffness (location, quality and extent) in your muscles, maintain this awareness as you gently and gradually move into the stretch, *thinking* first of releasing the tightness before you begin to move. *Don't force it.* Move a little, then stop, before you feel you're pushing too far, too fast. Give yourself time to become accustomed to each new stage in the movement before you take it further; this will enable you to persist without fear of hurting yourself.

Without forcing the stretch, try to *stay with* the new experience, in complete awareness of where you are and what it feels like. Establish a comfortable connection with where your body is now, stretch a little further—then stop. Move along the stretch a little further still—then stop. Always stop at the point where you feel that the stretch has gone as far as it wants to for now. Stay there for a moment. Think of breathing into the area you're working on. Then see if you can take the movement a little further. Approach each movement in an exploratory way—see what's going on, without judging yourself. And never, never force or yank. A slow, gentle but persistent release is what you want. If you feel you haven't gone far enough, be patient. Next time you will.

progress, your breaths will become longer and fuller. What is the feeling in your body as the breaths become easier? There will probably be an interplay: as the incoming and outgoing breaths become longer, fuller and deeper, your body releases more deeply, permitting the breaths to become still longer, fuller, deeper—and freer.

"GOOD" AND "BAD PAIN"

Some of these movements may be uncomfortable, perhaps even painful, at certain points—especially if you're very stiff and tight. Muscles that are being awakened perhaps for the first time in years may protest until they learn to like being released. If you try to pull back from the pain, or stiffen in dread of it, you'll defeat the purpose, which is *gently* and *gradually* to release the tightness that is the cause of the pain. *Never push, pull, yank or in any way force a movement.* If you reach a point of painful resistance, stop, tune in to exactly what you're feeling, try to stay with it or perhaps retreat a little, let your breath out (discomfort tends to make us hold our breath), let the breath

move in again, and resume. Try to *work through* the discomfort or tightness, rather than resisting or trying to circumvent it with a Creative Cheat (see next page).

Muscle cramps are your friends. They tell you where work is needed.

It's important to be able to distinguish between "good" and "bad" pain. "Good" pain is the pain of restoring elasticity to a tight muscle, which I teach my students to refer to as "release of tension." "Bad" pain is a serious message that warns of incipient injury. Any *sudden* shooting pain, any pain that feels like a dislocation or a twist, should bring you to a halt immediately. Check your Stance grid, with special attention to your knees, for meticulously correct alignment in the letter "H." Cautiously resume the movement, very gently and tentatively. If the pain persists or intensifies, stop. When you want to resume the movement, take some full breaths and proceed very carefully, checking to see if you are indeed "releasing tension" or actually hurting yourself; stop if you feel the warning pain.

PROCESS, NOT END RESULT

As you work your way through these movements, don't think of them as "exercises" to be done with as quickly as possible. Nor is it the number of repetitions ("reps") of the movements that matters; you'll find that in most cases very few reps are suggested. The point is the *quality of awareness* that you bring to each movement, not how intensely or how fast you do it. If you're directed (as in Movement #1) to hang down over your legs, letting the weight of your head pull your spine down, the purpose is not to get yourself down as far as possible as fast as possible, but rather to perform the movement with as much attentiveness as possible—and perhaps even as slowly as possible.

You'll learn to focus on a movement as you proceed with it, with the fullest possible awareness of what you're doing,

where you are, what you're experiencing *at the moment*, and not thinking of the goal— for the goal in these movements is the *awareness of the moment*. Above all, there should be no blind rushing toward the final position, thinking only of getting there.

If you keep your attention on what you're doing while you're doing it, instead of focusing on the thought of the final position, you'll find that your body will take increasing pleasure in these movements for their own sake. And this continuing act of attention as you proceed is far more important than how far you can go with any repetition. It's also the source of motivating yourself to continue, as you notice just where you are with no expectation.

First go through the whole set of movements systematically, from #1 to #34. Do each movement at least twice, as precisely as you can. The second time is usually much easier. After you've run through the entire series once or twice, begin to concentrate on a few movements that you feel address your problems. Often these are the ones that seem truly impossible, such as #18 (Ankle Sit) or #14

CREATIVE CHEATS

Some (or many!) of the movements will be difficult at first—that's why we're doing them. What is essential is that you not try to bypass the early discomfort with a Creative Cheat—an instant alternative chosen by your body/mind to avoid the prospect of pain as you stretch and release the tight places. A Creative Cheat lets you *look* as if you're doing a movement when in fact you've found a comfortable way of faking it. (I use the word "creative" because I'm always amazed at the mind's agility at figuring out shortcuts and ways of fooling ourselves.)

For example, in Movement #24 (Sitting Forward Bend), which gives a powerful stretch along the undersides of the legs and the lower and middle back, you're asked to sit with your legs straight out in front of you and bend forward at the hips so that eventually your whole torso extends out over your legs. At first you may scarcely be able to bend at all at the hips because your hamstrings and lower back muscles will be so tight; however, if you bend your legs at the knees, you can get your torso quite far down on the first try. This is a Creative Cheat that completely undermines the purpose of the movement. If you bend your knees, you are *flexing* your leg muscles, not *stretching* them. Your mind decides to avoid what it knows will hurt—the stretch up the legs. So it immediately switches to a close approximation, one that seems adequate but will not ask or allow your body to change.

Concentrate on the *process* of the movement, not the end result. The point of the movement is *not* to get your head down over your legs, but gradually to stretch the muscles of your legs and back. Getting your head down is only the end result—and it will happen automatically if you do the work of the stretch. Focus your breath directly into the place that feels tight and gently focus *through* it!

(Wrists on Railing). There will be days when you don't feel up to running through a good portion of the menu and will be tempted to do none at all. This is not an "all or nothing" routine; on those days, do just a few. You might want to make your own list of the ones that are hardest for you and make a point of doing those faithfully every day. (See Chapter Five for suggestions on how many movements to do, how often, and so on.)

Wear a bathing suit or leotard, or footless tights or leggings and a shirt—anything that allows your legs to be perfectly seen. Shorts are fine, provided they don't bind you at the crotch. Bare feet are essential. Don't wear shoes, or socks, or tights with feet. Your feet must be free and should make direct contact with the floor.

Each movement is designed to locate and focus on a place where you're likely to be tight and/or weak—so welcome the feedback. Let yourself *feel* what there is to feel. Breathe. Feel some more. Know that you *will* see and feel improvement, often after doing the Stance and the Thirty-Four Movements for the first time.

DRIVING FOR SUCCESS

BILL'S STORY

I wasn't sure at first how much I'd be able to help Bill, a man of thirty-eight who drove long hours at a stretch to cover his sales route in the West. He had back pain that was difficult to relieve because he was forced to maintain the position that made it worse: sitting hunched over the wheel of his car. But he had started with bad posture in the first place—a swayback and bowlegs that increased the pressure on his lower back. He sat either too far back over his hips, so that his spine was stressed by squeezed-together abdominals, or with a swayback, which compressed the muscles of his lower back.

Over a period of months we worked together whenever he was in town, concentrating on lengthening his back and strengthening his abdominal muscles. Eventually we were able to give him a natural "girdle" formed by the muscles of his whole lower torso—strong abdominals and back muscles that held him firmly and made it possible for him to sit easily upright even during his many hours on the road. And of course he learned to get out and take a good stretch whenever he had to stop for gas, or whenever he got tired or felt pain and tension coming on.

By learning to listen attentively to feedback from his body, and taking a stretch or a rest before the trouble became acute, Bill no longer found driving long distances an ordeal. He arrived at his destinations feeling fresh and energetic, not worn out from pain and fatigue.

THE VANCE STANCE

Lengthens neck and spine; releases tension by letting the weight of the head gently pull down, separating the vertebrae

POSITION

Assume the Stance (first running through it point by point). Then let your head drop gently forward on your neck. Let your arms hang loose, and be sure your knees are deeply bent. When your head is hanging down as long on your neck as possible, start to roll down your spine, vertebra by vertebra. Use your head as a weight in this gentle pull. Pause at each new setting to allow your neck to lengthen out again.

Be sure that your ankles, knees and hips are bent. Feel the weight of your body settle down into your legs as you continue to roll down, until the palms of your hands brush or rest on the floor. Your legs are well hinged at the ankles, knees and hips, your spine is stretched long, your neck is very long, and your weight is centered over your feet. Remember to let your breath move freely in and out, exhaling on an "S."

To come back up, flex even more deeply at the ankles and knees, then roll your spine up, vertebra by vertebra. Continue to let your head hang on a long neck until you get up as far as the shoulders, then let your head lift up over your neck.

Keep your weight centered over your feet to hold the PIECE OF PAPER in place.

Roll down very slowly, feeling the release along your spine.

Don't worry if at first your hands don't reach the floor. They will, once you've released the tension in your neck and spine.

OBJECT

Consciously to release the neck and the spine, allowing the downward pull of gravity on the head to lengthen the neck and spine, vertebra by vertebra; to experience the gentle letting-go pull of gravity all the way down the spine and into the legs.

NOTICE

How much tension is there in the back of your neck? Think of breathing "into" your neck (i.e., in your imagination, direct the flow of breath into your neck) and into each vertebra of your spine as it drops longer and longer. You should feel a release of tension at each point where you breathe into your neck and spine.

IF THIS IS IMPOSSIBLE

Be sure you're not asking yourself to "touch your toes." This is not the point of the movement; we just want your head to drop down so that you hang over like a rag doll, giving in completely to the pull of gravity. Your job is only to drop your head, let go all along your spine, keep your joints well flexed, and *breathe*. Be sure your weight remains well centered over your feet even in this upside-down position, and that your heels are planted well down on the floor (holding down the PIECE OF PAPER).

IF THIS IS EASY

Pay special attention to any tension in the back of your neck; make sure your neck continues to release and lengthen as you hang lower and lower, longer and longer. It's tempting to contract the back of your neck in reaction to the strangeness of the new sensations produced by allowing your spine to release freely. Keep checking that your neck is free. Breathe, release a little further, pause—and continue. (In the future, you can do this as part of Movement #2.)

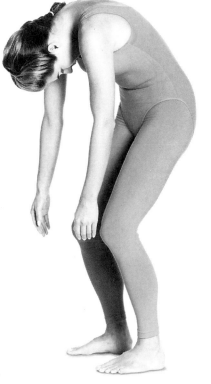

When rolling up, keep your head down. Only after you've pulled your body upright should your neck and head return to their original positions.

THE VANCE STANCE

Stretches hamstrings, calves and Achilles tendons

POSITION

With your body dropped down and hanging easily, as in Movement #1 but with your arms slightly farther in front of you, place the palms of your hands flat on the floor, shoulder-width apart, with your fingers pointing straight ahead. Straighten one leg at a time, keeping your heels pressed well down. Release, and repeat with the other leg.

OBJECT

To stretch the backs of the legs (the hamstring muscles, calves and Achilles tendons) while keeping the hands flat on the floor, feet pointing straight ahead and heels in contact with the floor.

NOTICE

Is one leg tighter up the back than the other, or is one foot turned out more than the other? This often happens on the same side where back pain occurs. It's as though the tightness in the leg extends all the way up your back, pulling it tight on that side, to compensate for the shortness of the leg muscles.

Your hands should be flat on the floor with your fingers pointing straight ahead. Straighten one leg, keeping the other bent with the heel pressed down.

Straighten the other leg while releasing the opposite leg.

IF THIS IS IMPOSSIBLE

Be content just to get your hands and feet on the floor at the same time. Your legs can be bent if necessary, and your feet as far apart as needed. Now straighten one leg, keeping the heel down. Release. Straighten the other leg. Feel the stretch up the back of each leg: in the Achilles tendon (from the ankle to the calf) and hamstring (back of the knee up the leg to the buttocks). At what points do you feel locked or "frozen"? Make sure your head hangs loose throughout the movement; keep releasing the back of your neck.

IF THIS IS EASY

Straighten both legs at the same time, pressing the base of your spine up as your heels go down.

NOTICE

Are your legs equally flexible? Or must you "correct" to become symmetrical—is one side more difficult to straighten than the other? Hold the position for about six full breaths (on the "S" exhale). Make sure both heels are pressing down firmly into the floor.

To get back up, flex deeply at ankles and knees, and roll up your spine, vertebra by vertebra, as in Movement #1.

When this movement becomes easy, straighten both legs at the same time, keeping your heels down. Be sure your neck is released and your head hangs down, centered between your arms.

3 DOORWAY STRETCH

Stretches across chest; opens and frees shoulder joints; flattens upper back ("dowager's hump")

POSITION

Stand facing an open doorway, with your feet just a little back from the center of the door frame. Place your arms on the wall to either side of the door frame (or on the frame itself) so that the upper arm and the forearm make a right angle. Palms are flat against the wall, as are upper arms and forearms; shoulders are back and down, and in line with the elbows. Think yourself into the alignment of the Stance (legs, torso and head). How does this alignment affect the position you're in now?

Imagine that the GOLDEN HOOK at the top of your head is centered under the overhead frame and that your head wants to rise up to attach to the frame and hang down from it, stretching your neck long. Now lean slightly forward, directing the stretch *out* through your elbows as well.

OBJECT

To release tightness in shoulders and arms, using the wall or door frame as passive resistance. Applying external pressure on the shoulders and back, stretching across the chest and arms and contracting the back of the arms will gently open the shoulder joints. Bracing the arms and leaning slightly forward will encourage a stretch across the shoulder girdle as the back contracts.

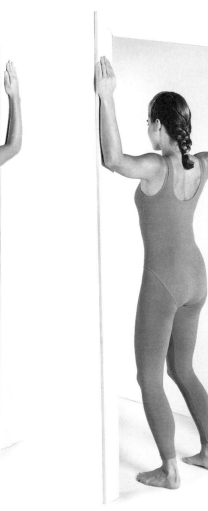

Be sure your head is centered in the door frame and your weight falls evenly on both feet.

Keeping the Stance, lean your body slightly forward. Drop your shoulders and do not let your neck shorten as you lean forward.

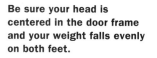

NOTICE

Does your neck shorten as you lean forward or try to press your shoulders down? It is essential to uncover and correct this automatic habit in order to keep your neck free of your shoulders, able to lengthen freely regardless of shoulder and arm movement. Feel the deep stretch in the front of your shoulders. It may be very uncomfortable. Stretch gently, gradually, and breathe into the release. Try to keep your neck long as you widen and *drop* your shoulders.

IF THIS IS IMPOSSIBLE

Try the movement first with just one arm. Place the arm out as low as necessary on the wall to begin to be comfortable as you start to drop that shoulder. Then

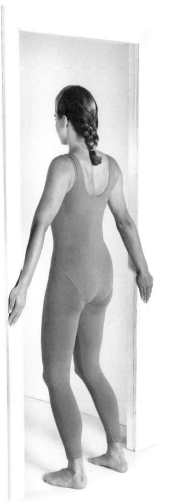

Until this movement becomes easy, start with your hands lower down on the door frame; in time, you'll be able to begin with your elbows bent and your arms at right angles.

add the other arm, gradually moving your hands wider and higher with your elbows down, more in line with your shoulders, as you begin to open up your shoulder joints and arms.

IF THIS IS EASY

Make sure your shoulders are quite strongly pressed down from within, and that you keep lengthening your neck. Don't let the small of your back push forward into a swayback.

ADVANCED VERSION

Extend your arms straight up overhead, elbows straight and shoulders down. Be sure to lock the elbow joints as you drop your shoulders.

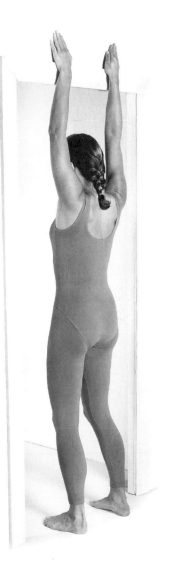

Keep your elbow joints locked as you lower your shoulders and lean forward.

4

ARMS BEHIND ON RAILING

Opens arms;
stretches
shoulders;
opens front of
chest

POSITION

Standing with your back up against a railing (or barre) or the edge of an open door, use both hands to grasp the railing or doorknobs behind you with an overhand grip. Walk about eighteen inches away from the railing or door, assume the Stance and lean slightly farther away from it. With your hands firmly gripping the railing or knob, straighten your elbows. Tuck your pelvis under and lean farther into the stretch, keeping your knees flexed. Drop your shoulders back and down (push them down if necessary), keeping your elbows straight, your neck long and your head up. Work on *relaxing* your shoulders, back and down, and straightening your elbows.

OBJECT

To stabilize the hands and keep the arms locked straight so that the stretch will come in the shoulders, with leverage pushing them back and down; also, to open up the front of the chest and tighten the slack area across the back.

Plant your heels on the floor to hold down the PIECE OF PAPER.

Whether using a railing or door, be sure to keep both arms the same distance from your body, elbows straight, neck long and head up.

NOTICE

Be aware of how the position of your feet affects where you feel the stretch. Experiment with how far away from the railing or door you must stand in order to get a contraction in your upper back and *not* in your lower back, making you swaybacked.

IF THIS IS IMPOSSIBLE

Grasp the railing or knob with one hand at a time. Feel what is keeping you from being able to lock your arm at the elbow; it may be deep tightness in that arm (above and/or below the elbow) that is unused to allowing energy to flow through it. Exhale as you think of the tightness flowing down and out the arm. Do the other arm. Then do the movement with both hands. If using a railing, place your hands far apart at first, gradually bringing them closer as the movement becomes easier.

IF THIS IS EASY

Imagine yourself as the figurehead on the prow of a ship, wind blowing at your back, and expand your chest as you become fuller and more open at the front. Ah! Feels nice, doesn't it? Be sure to keep lengthening your neck, and don't let the small of your back push forward.

Do this movement with each arm until it becomes possible to do it with both arms at once.

5

HEEL DROP ON STAIRS

Stretches
Achilles
tendons;
increases flexion
in ankle joints

POSITION

Facing a flight of stairs, stand on the bottom step. Plant your toes and the balls of your feet firmly on the step and let your heels hang down off the edge as you hold on to the banister or wall. Think your way up the Stance, but keep your feet *together* instead of hip-width apart.

OBJECT

To allow the weight of the body to stretch the Achilles tendons and to open the ankle joints. *Remember, the ankle is a crucial joint upon which everything else depends.* If it cannot flex and extend freely, you will compensate for this limitation all the way up your body and your range of movement will be restricted throughout. Keep your heels pushed down well below the edge of the step, with your pelvis tucked under and knees bent. Do not bounce.

NOTICE

Thinking yourself into the Stance, with your feet together instead of apart, do you find yourself cheating at any point? Are you pushing your hips out too far to the back or side because your Achilles tendons are too tight to permit a stretch? Or are you maintaining good alignment as you stretch your Achilles tendons, however much or little you can?

IF THIS IS IMPOSSIBLE

If you're unable to do this movement, it's because you're very tight in the Achilles tendons, ankle joints or shins. After you've practiced #18 (Ankle Sit), which stretches the front of the foot and extends the ankle joint, try it again.

Drive your feet down at an angle as far as possible with your heels pushed down.

IF THIS IS EASY

As you continue to drop your heels, bend your knees further as you press down; feel the contraction all the way up the front of your foot and leg.

ADVANCED VERSION

Let one leg take all your weight, allowing the other to remain on the step but go loose. Feel how this increases the intensity of the Achilles stretch and allows more contraction up the front of the leg. Change legs and repeat, maintaining the Stance even

though your weight is on one leg.

Come off the steps and assume the Stance again. Notice how much easier it is now as the places where you felt tight and stiff—the shoulders, the back, the neck and the legs—begin to release.

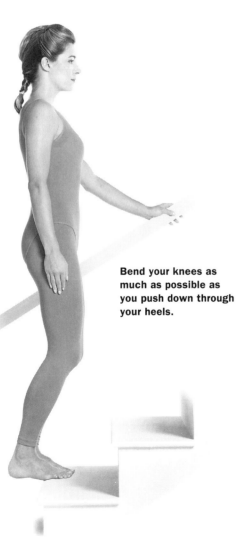

Bend your knees as much as possible as you push down through your heels.

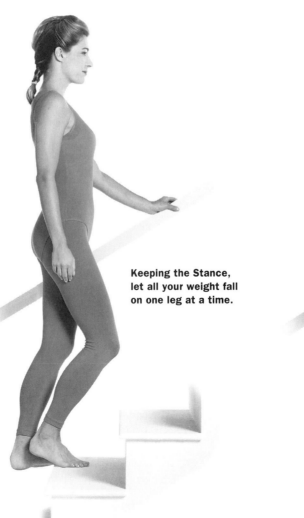

Keeping the Stance, let all your weight fall on one leg at a time.

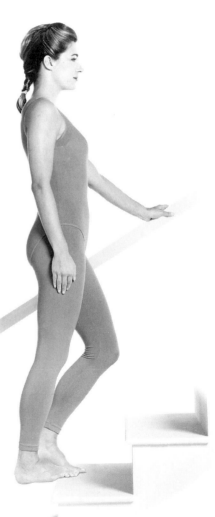

Indicates where the spine has been shortened; lengthens back muscles from hips to neck

POSITION

Stand with your back against a wall and your feet about fourteen inches out from it, knees bent so that your thighs and lower legs form almost a ninety-degree angle. Press the small of your back flat against the wall, keeping your upper back flat against the wall at the same time and the back of your head touching it. Hold your arms away from your sides and place the backs of your hands against the wall.

OBJECT

To flatten the whole back, as well as the back of the head, against the wall by using the pressure of the feet on the floor. (Your neck will still curve slightly inward, away from the wall. This is a natural curve.)

NOTICE

Feel the interconnection between the small of your back and your neck. Does it seem impossible to flatten your back while keeping the back of your head against the wall? Does your neck tend to shorten with the effort of trying to keep your head against the wall? Does your lower back tilt forward into a swayback as you press your head against the wall? This is symptomatic of a shortened spine—one part has to curve in order to keep another part flat.

IF THIS IS IMPOSSIBLE

Concentrate on getting the small of your back against the wall. Walk your feet out from the wall as far as necessary, until you can tilt your pelvis back to press your waist flat. Don't worry if at first your head drops forward and your shoulders have to round slightly to achieve this. You must be able to feel what it means to have contact there; then gradually add the length in the spine.

Be sure that your upper back is flat against the wall and that the back of your head touches the wall as well.

Your feet can be as far away from the wall as necessary to get the small of your back against the wall.

STANCE CHECK

Rethink the Stance in this movement. Check your feet (pointing straight ahead), ankles (rolling neither inward nor outward) and knees (HEADLIGHTS beaming straight ahead). Let the RACCOON EYES at your hip joints open wider. Does this help you get more of the small of your back against the wall? Remember that the answer to every problem is to think *more length*. Is your PAIL OF WATER level? Are you making enough space to receive the SHIMS as you insert them one by one? Is the PLUNGER sticking straight out in front? Is your neck long and relaxed? Is the GOLDEN HOOK extending straight up from the center of the top of your head?

IF THIS IS EASY

Maintaining the same alignment as when you are flat against the wall, push yourself away from the wall with your fingertips. Stand in the Stance, feeling those subtle connections allowed by aligning your back along the wall.

ADVANCED VERSION

In the basic position, with your back to the wall, place your arms flat against the wall so that the upper arms from shoulder to elbow are parallel to the floor and the forearms are perpendicular—as in "You're under arrest!" Feel where the effort is to keep everything flat and long—neck, upper back, middle of back, small of back. Don't let your neck shorten; concentrate on continuing to lengthen it as you drop your shoulders further.

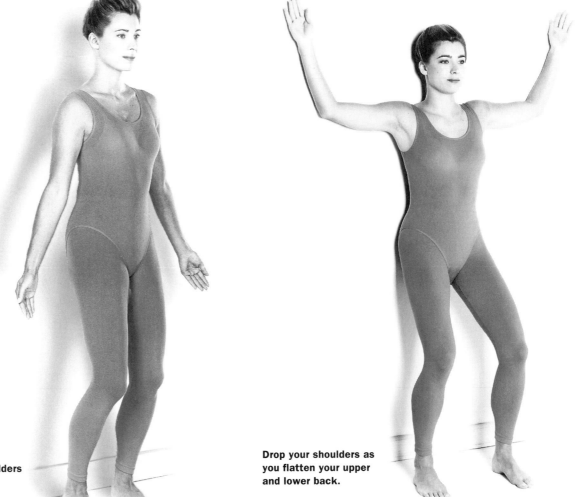

Make sure your shoulders are back and down.

Drop your shoulders as you flatten your upper and lower back.

THE VANCE STANCE

Stretches one side of the torso while contracting the muscles of the opposite side

POSITION

Stand in the Stance, with your feet a little more than shoulder-width apart. Let your right arm hang down along your right thigh, and press your hand into your leg for support. Drop your head to the right, raising your left arm straight up overhead. On an "S"-exhale, lean to the right and drop your head to that side, curving your raised (left) arm over your head to the right as your right arm slides farther down your thigh. Feel the stretch all along your waist and out through your arm.

Exhale, being sure to press both heels into the floor. Release, and repeat on the other side.

OBJECT

To stretch the muscles along the sides of the torso (the obliques) by arcing the upper body sideways, simultaneously contracting the muscles of the opposite side, in order to make the torso both strong and flexible (and to make it easier to lift as the SHIMS are inserted in the Stance).

Roll your ankles out as your feet move wider in the Stance.

Once you stretch the muscles along your torso, you'll be able to reach farther and lower with the raised arm.

Stretch as far to the side as you can without bending forward or arching your back.

NOTICE

Is there pain in the small of your back? If so, you're leaning too far back and putting pressure there. Watch that you're neither bending forward, leading with your head or shoulder, nor bending backwards, stressing the small of your back. Go *straight* over to the side, as if your whole body were being flattened between two panes of glass.

IF THIS IS IMPOSSIBLE

Begin by raising your arm and hand only, and just dropping your head to the other side. Breathe into the tight place, and wait. When the tightness eases, let the other arm press firmly into the leg, increasing the degree of lean.

IF THIS IS EASY

Watch yourself in the mirror as you try to form a smooth, scythe-shaped curve with one side of your body. Your neck should be relaxed, your head hanging easily to the same side. (In other words, if you're stretching to the right, your head hangs over to the right—but facing squarely front.) The hip of the opposite leg should press slightly out to the side as you extend your top arm and pull over in the opposite direction. Reach out with the raised arm, straightening the elbow, and try to touch an imaginary wall on the far side. Press down firmly into the heel of your left foot so that the stretch extends all the way down into the leg on that side.

STANCE CHECK

Make sure your buttocks stay firmly tucked under as you bend sideways and that the PAIL OF WATER doesn't tip toward the front.

ADVANCED VERSION

From the very long and stretched basic position, lift the other arm up to meet the top (left) arm. Press your palms together and reach still farther out to the side. Release. Reverse the movement, with the right side stretching to the left. This stretch lengthens the muscles of the waist and midriff, helping to reduce "spare tires." Do the stretch with both arms overhead only after the first version has become very easy.

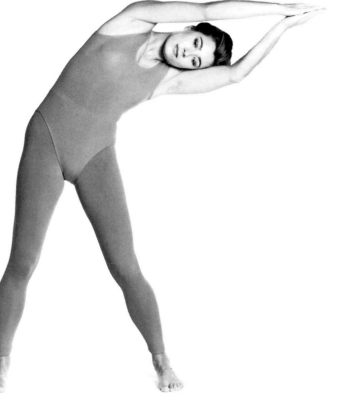

Press strongly down on the outside of the foot opposite to the direction of the lean in order to anchor yourself to the floor.

THE VANCE STANCE

For balance: increases the stretch along the fronts of the thighs and hip joints; contracts and strengthens lower legs and feet

POSITION

Assume the Stance, lifting strongly in your upper body as you keep your heels firmly planted on the floor. Now lift and grasp one leg at the knee, pulling it in toward your chest with both hands. Lace your fingers around the knee for a better grip as you balance on one leg.

Repeat on the other side.

OBJECT

To rise up and remain standing tall and balanced on one leg with the other drawn in toward the chest, contracting (closing) the RACCOON EYE of the raised leg and stretching (opening) the RACCOON EYE of the standing leg; also, to keep the back long and straight, even when the raised leg pulls in.

NOTICE

Do you find yourself bending over in an attempt to balance? Does the standing leg want to bend to make it easier to pull the other leg toward you? Both these Creative Cheats are attempts to get into the position (standing on one leg) without using the correct muscles—those of the front thigh of the standing leg and the hip flexors of the

As you pull the bent leg into your chest, be sure not to round your back or tilt to the side.

bending leg, as well as those of the back. Pay particular attention also to the muscles of the foot, arch and outside lower leg; these muscles will be working very hard if you're correctly aligned, especially if you have bowlegs or knock-knees. Keep tall, and try not to resort to a Creative Cheat. Keep the pressure applied directly to the demands of the position; don't allow it to be deflected.

IF THIS IS IMPOSSIBLE

Is it the balancing that's giving you trouble, or do you find it difficult to pull your leg up and in? Begin by leaning sideways against a wall, for stability. Then, holding yourself up, lean slowly away from the wall.

STANCE CHECK

Feel how you must be tilted much more forward than usual to be in the energy stream. Press down on the PIECE OF PAPER with your heel to keep from toppling forward. Lift your toes for a moment to send the pressure back to your heel even more firmly.

ADVANCED VERSION

Let your arms relax at your sides and, with your knee up, extend your leg. Imagine that a balloon is tied to your knee to keep it aloft. Pointing your toes, lightly flick your lower leg straight out,

then back in, keeping your knee as high as possible. Maintain a tall, erect torso. *Think the two-way energy stream.* Feel how it keeps your torso tall and straight, so that you don't bend over or slump back in the effort to extend your leg.

Advanced version: Unclasp your hands and let the raised leg form a right angle.

When flicking your lower leg, try to keep the top of that leg steady from knee to hip and your torso rising straight up from your pelvis.

9

TOE CRUNCH SERIES (I)

Releases tightness in undersides of toes (especially good for bunions and hammertoes); stretches front of foot, increasing extension of ankle joint; strengthens Achilles tendon

LIFT FOOT TO SQUARED-OFF TOES

POSITION

Stand behind the back of a chair (or next to a table or barre), holding on to the back for support. Bend your right foot at the toes, lifting the heel but keeping the toes on the floor. Your knee is bent. The heel and arch of your foot are lined up over your toes, not dropped outward or inward.

Repeat on the other side.

OBJECT

To get the foot to form a complete right angle with the toes; also, to release, through gentle pressure, tightness of the undersides of the toes and the arch of the foot, and to stretch the front of the foot and contract the Achilles tendon by raising the heel.

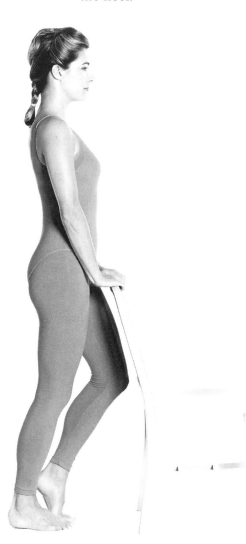

Try to form a right angle with your toes and the rest of your foot as you press forward with your raised heel. Don't let your toes grip the floor.

Your weight should be divided equally over both feet.

NOTICE

Are your toes curled under like a parrot's claws? Do they form a pyramid shape at the pads? Do they feel as if they might break off if you bend them? These are signs of an immobilizing tightness and stiffness in the toe muscles and joints, whose elasticity must be restored to gain access to the rest of your body.

Do you feel a pull, perhaps under your toes or directly upon the big-toe joint? This exercise is important and should be done daily if you have bunions and/or hammertoes, which means that this area is very tight and contracted. You will feel some strong discomfort with the release, perhaps even some pain. Be very gentle but persistent as you do this movement. Keep the pressure mild and steady; don't jerk or pull.

Press your heel forward as you keep your toes flat on the floor, breathing into them.

IF THIS IS IMPOSSIBLE

Reach down and lengthen your toes with your hands, pulling them out straight as far as they'll go. *Concentrate on not gripping with your toes* as you start to press your heel forward. Stand up and focus on where the discomfort is. Breathe into it. As it eases, gently press the instep forward, eventually forming a right angle at the toes.

IF THIS IS EASY

Make sure your toes are really flat, not curling under at all as you bend the joint. Check that all toenails are facing upward. Press your heel straight forward, as far as possible, keeping it in line laterally as well as front to back. Make your toes hinge squarely.

ADVANCED VERSION

From this bent-toe position, with your foot lined up over your toes, put your weight on the ledge that you've made with them. Keep your knee bent. Lift your other foot off the floor, balancing on one foot (and using the chair,

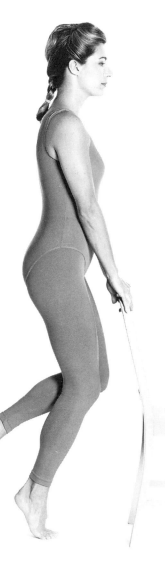

Keeping your PAIL OF WATER level, put your weight on the ledge you've made with your toes.

table or barre). Exhale on an "S," then let the breath come in. If you can, maintain this position for about three complete breaths. Come down off your toes.

Don't worry if you have trouble keeping your balance or can't lift the standing leg off the ground. The body and mind are so intertwined that the slightest doubt that you might not be able to stand in this new way signals your brain to play it safe and not even try. Hold on more firmly to the chair (or table or barre) and push down with your hands to gain confidence in your ability to balance. Try again. This may take a while if your toes are very cramped and stiff.

THE VANCE STANCE

Stretches shin, top of foot and toes; contracts arch

BEND FOOT OVER, OPEN SHIN

POSITION

From the same starting position as before (standing behind a chair, table or barre), lift your foot and flip your toes over so there is a gentle pressure along the top of your foot and toes. Press into your ankle from behind, folding your toes under as you stretch along your shin and the top of your foot. Pressing your heel forward from behind, aim at forming a straight line with the front of your leg and your foot. Keep your foot and heel in straight vertical alignment, not allowing the heel to drop out to one side. Feel the powerful stretch up the front of your foot, which increases as the heel presses forward. This movement can be very uncomfortable if you have foot problems, since it stretches an area that has long been tight. If you persist, it will soon begin to feel good—a welcome releasing stretch.

Repeat on the other side.

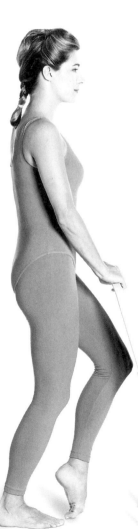

With your toes folded under, press your raised heel forward.

When you do the movements with each foot, you might find that one is more flexible than the other.

OBJECT

To reverse the normal position of the foot and ankle, from a right angle to a straight line, releasing the tightness that causes foot problems in toes, arches, shins and Achilles tendons; also, to allow the arch to contract for more strength.

NOTICE

Do you feel as if the front of your foot and/or leg might actually break off? This is normal and will ease if you persist with the movement.

IF THIS IS IMPOSSIBLE

Practice just holding your foot in this position, with the heel raised and the toes *beginning* to fold under. Don't try to stretch further. Reduce the stretch to the point where you can tolerate the discomfort up the front of your leg. We are trying to lengthen the entire front of the lower leg and foot, increasing the intensity of the stretch by folding the toes under. Your legs and feet were designed to be able to bend this way (however unlikely it seems now), and with time and patience it will become easy.

IF THIS IS EASY

Press your heel all the way forward, so that your foot and leg form a straight line in front.

ADVANCED VERSION

With your toes still folded under, gently drop your heel toward the floor as if your toenails were set in concrete. As your heel approaches the floor, bend that knee even further to increase the stretch in the foot. If you get a cramp in your toes or arch, welcome it as a positive sign that you're giving your foot a much-needed stretch, extending its flexibility. *Cramps are your friends!* Reverse the position to ease the cramp, then continue.

Try to stand on that foot with the toes still folded under and the knee and ankle very deeply bent, feeling the full weight of your body through the entire leg and foot, stretching the foot and shin out from within.

"BAD FEET"

Our feet are so vital to everything that happens above them, and their "work area" is so amazingly small, that they cannot afford the slightest distortion or interference. As it is, however, most fashionable shoes narrow toward the toes, squeezing them together, forcing the big toe out of alignment—and causing foot problems for literally millions of women. Few of us, in fact, have not suffered some degree of deformity: bunions, hammertoes, corns, calluses.

Just try on a pair of shoes with good toe room and you'll immediately feel your toes expanding to fill the space provided by the footbed. Even running shoes are much better for your feet than "street" shoes, although these too tend to narrow somewhat in the toes. I advise my women clients to buy men's tennis shoes, which are cut wider across the toes, and to get the largest size they can wear. Among the worst offenders are thong sandals: in order to keep them on, you have to grip with the four outer toes, virtually immobilizing the ankle and causing great tension and tightness all the way up the leg.

I urge all women to take responsibility for the well-being of their own feet by choosing shoes that allow the foot to spread out as it wants to in walking. This means shoes that are flat, preferably with a strap, and cut wide across the toes. (Birkenstocks are ideal.) Only this type of shoe can put an end to our complaints of "bad feet."

Releases
tightness in
muscles of
foot (top and
bottom) from
heel to toes;
opens legs

POSITION

Assume the Stance sideways to a railing or the back of a chair. Holding on to the railing or chair, place a tennis ball directly beneath the center of your heel. Put most of your weight on the ball, as if to press it down

through the floor. Exhale, and release any tension you find there. Now move the ball under your foot from the heel to the next setting, just in front of the heel. Repeat the releasing there. Move the ball to the middle of the arch. Release. Finally, move

the ball to the fourth setting, just under the toe joints, and release.

Repeat three or four times at each of the four settings, then switch to the other foot. Be sure to keep very upright as you maintain the Stance with both knees well bent.

This movement consists of four settings for each foot. a) Pin the ball under the heel of your foot. b) Move the ball to just in front of your heel, then c) to the middle of the arch and d) to under the toe joints.

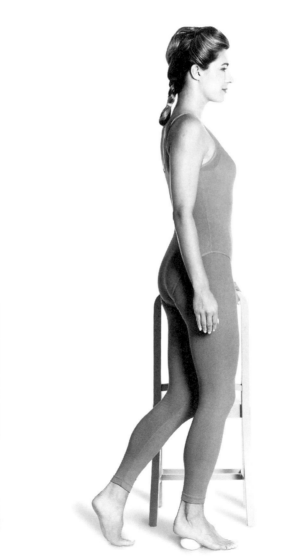

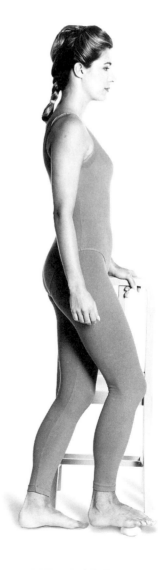

OBJECT

To use the pressure and weight of the leg and foot on the ball to open up tight places in the feet, legs and thighs.

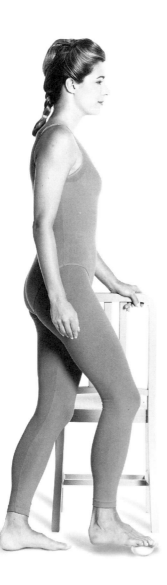

NOTICE

This may feel extremely tight and painful. Particularly if you have back or foot trouble, you are likely to have great tightness deep in the muscles of the foot and leg. Does it seem impossible that you could ever place enough weight on your foot to be actually "standing" on it with the ball underneath? This is quite common in people whose spines are shortened and contracted, and who are not allowing their feet and legs to do the work they were designed for.

IF THIS IS IMPOSSIBLE

First concentrate on maintaining the Stance (or even *attempting* to get your body to try it!) while you simply rest your foot lightly on the ball at the first setting, under the heel. Exhale, at the same time paying attention to where it hurts and where you might be feeling the beginning of release—where the rigidity of the foot muscles may start to soften and the muscles become mobile again. Then move to each next setting, allowing your breath to begin to open there. Notice which one is the most painful. Gradually, you'll be able to do at least two settings with comfort. The rest will follow. Keep much of your weight on your supporting leg until the muscles of the working foot begin to release.

IF THIS IS EASY

Increase the pressure on your foot as it opens at each setting, from heel to toes. When the tennis ball is just behind the ball of your foot, where the toes join the foot, press your heel down while you bend the ankle and knee, and curve your foot all along the curve of the ball. This gives a powerful stretch to the top of the foot, the toe joints, the arch and the ankle. As the muscles of your foot release, feel the corresponding release up through your leg. You may tremble or shake, especially if you're heavy-set, as your leg comes alive. Keep breathing through it, and continue.

11

MONKEY WALK

Stretches muscles along outside and top of foot; strengthens arch

POSITION

Assume the Stance. Roll your ankles and feet all the way to the outside, curling your toes under and aiming the HEADLIGHTS of your knees out to the side, angled off away from each other. Imagine that you are an ape at the beach, scooping up sand with your curled-under toes and feet. Walk about a little, maintaining the gripped feet and very bent knees.

OBJECT

To stretch the muscles along the outside and top of the foot, and to contract and strengthen the arch to better support the foot. This will make it much easier to stand in the Stance with your feet pointing straight ahead rather than turned out.

NOTICE

If you get a cramp in your foot as you do this movement, you're on your way! This is what we want to happen. We want energy to reach areas that have been blocked, and cramps signify an awareness of the blocking. Think of directing your breath into the place where you feel the discomfort; release the cramp by coming out of the movement, stretching your toes upward, off the floor, in the opposite direction. When the cramp is relieved, resume the folded-under position and continue.

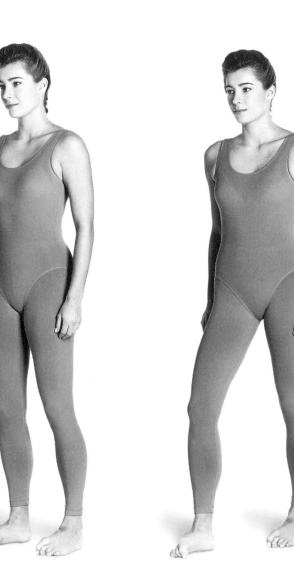

Rest your weight on the outsides of your feet and curl your toes under. Maintain this posture as you walk around the room. Notice how much your pelvis and knees want to lock in order to avoid opening the muscles down the legs and in the feet.

IF THIS IS IMPOSSIBLE

It may be difficult for you to get your toes to curl under at all, or it may seem impossible to put your full weight on your foot with the toes curled. The big toe, especially, may not bend enough. This is to be expected if you have foot problems or back trouble: tight feet affect many other areas of the body. Do #5 (Heel Drop on Stairs) and #18 (Ankle Sit) as often as possible, and do the Monkey Walk as best you can for now. Your feet will gradually gain in flexibility if you persist.

IF THIS IS EASY

Concentrate on bending more at the ankle and increasing the curl in the arch and the toes. Really *grip* with the toes. Tuck your pelvis well under, and drive your weight down the thigh into your foot as you stand on each leg in turn. Do the Monkey Walk as slowly as you can, as if in a slow-motion film sequence. Feel whether you're keeping the weight off your foot by straightening your knee, a Creative Cheat to avoid pain. If you are, think of sinking down with each step; try not to resist or brace yourself against the discomfort. If this is too painful, do just a little at a time, and think of consciously breathing into the tight area. Hold on to a table, chair or wall and try to allow that tight area to give a little. Consciously relaxing the rest of your body will help, too. When your feet are less tight, the movement will become much easier and begin to feel like an enjoyable stretch.

STANCE CHECK

Notice what parts of your body fall out of alignment when faced with such deep discomfort. The PAIL OF WATER may tip forward, the PLUNGER handle may drop and your knees may straighten. This instinctive misalignment comes from trying to protect yourself from going through the uncomfortable process of opening up your feet. Try to *go through* the discomfort, rather than resisting and avoiding it. Do everything super-slowly, stopping often and breathing into the tight or painful places. Resume when you can—but don't give up. You should feel results quite soon if you persist gently, staying with it. The pain is an indication of how tight you are and how much you need this movement.

LEARNING HOW TO WALK

You may think you already know how to walk—after all, you've been doing it most of your life. But, as with every other type of physical performance, there may be a more elegant or economical way. If you've experienced pain in walking or running, if you've noticed a gradual deterioration in your performance and you're starting to "walk like an old person," it is imperative that we identify the problem and correct it, substituting a new, more graceful and efficient means of locomotion.

The Monkey Walk and Groucho Walk are two extreme, artificial, practice ways to open your feet and legs so you can put the Stance into action. As with the Down-the-Stairs movement, the correct way is to go slowly with deeply bent ankles and knees, maintaining the bend all the way through the step, not lifting up or locking the knee at any time. This allows the torso to remain upright, not collapsed in the middle.

If this new way feels wrong, it's probably right. What you've been doing all your life naturally feels correct, like *you*, so the real right way will feel strange and unnatural at first. We are penetrating to the heart of your control system, attempting to unscramble crossed signals that go far back in your life. Have patience with your own first awkward steps in this new way. Do not judge yourself. After all, no one criticized your first clumsy attempts to walk. Be as gentle with yourself now, as indulgent, as your parents were with you then. Be your own loving parent!

12

Stretches
Achilles
tendons;
releases ankle
and hip joints;
stretches small
of back

POSITION

Assume the Stance, with your feet wider than hip-width apart. Keeping your heels *firmly planted,* drop your buttocks down as you sink into a deep squat, reaching your arms out between your knees.

OBJECT

To stretch the small of the back after releasing the hip and ankle joints by stretching the Achilles tendons, which is achieved by the extreme ankle flexion of the squatting position; also, to move the legs in and out freely while in the squatting position.

NOTICE

Do you tend to fall backwards? Or do you have trouble even getting down into a full squat? Many people with bad backs are so tight in the hips and lower back that they can't hinge enough to get into a squatting position. Do you tend to rise up on the balls of your feet, rather than hinging properly at the ankle, knee and hip joints so that you can keep your feet flat on the floor?

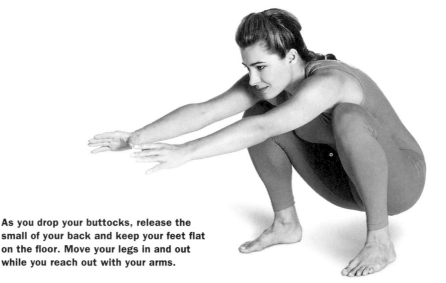

As you drop your buttocks, release the small of your back and keep your feet flat on the floor. Move your legs in and out while you reach out with your arms.

IF THIS IS IMPOSSIBLE

Grasp the sides of an open doorway or a sturdy railing with both hands, holding on as you walk yourself back and slowly lower yourself. Stop at the point where your heels start to lift, and press them down firmly. Lock your arms out straight. If you need to turn your feet out slightly (letting your heels move toward each other a little), that's okay. Do whatever you have to do with the rest of your body in order to press your heels flat on the floor.

Tune in to exactly where you're feeling the demands of this position (squatting) in your

body. Experiment with letting go first with one hand, then the other, then both, so that you're *reaching out* in front of you while squatting, with your heels down and keeping your balance.

IF THIS IS EASY

With your heels flat on the floor, reach your arms through your legs as far as you can. Relax your neck and shoulders; exhale as you slowly move your knees in and out, reaching more and more forward, pressing your heels down especially on the outside.

ADVANCED VERSION

From the squat, raise your buttocks until your legs and torso form a right angle. Flatten your back, and reach your arms out. Lower, and repeat. Make sure your knees stay directly out over your feet and don't drop to the inside as you come up.

A PIVOTAL POINT

As a major joint, the hip is often an area of much confusion and tightness. It is the point at which the energy stream divides to flow down through the legs and up through the torso. For energy moving downward, the hip joint reflects the condition of the ankles— if they are tight, the hips probably are, too. For energy moving up-ward, the hip is the gate-way to the back and must be released in order to free the back and the whole upper body.

People often try to force the hip joints open by pushing out at the knees. The hips can be released only in relation to the opening of the ankles and the lifting of the back. Each area in turn releases and opens the other.

Be sure your feet are flat on the floor.

Flatten your back as you stretch out your arms.

13

LEG ON RAILING

Stretches hamstrings, as well as front of thigh and hip and ankle of standing leg; also stretches back

POSITION

Stand facing a railing (or countertop or desk) about waist high. Lift one leg and place your heel on the railing in front of you but angled out to the side. (The back of the heel bone, not the Achilles tendon, should be touching.) The foot on the floor should be slightly turned out, at the same angle, to the opposite side. Gradually straighten both legs. Drop the hip of the raised leg to keep the PAIL OF WATER level, especially side to side.

Keep your buttocks tucked under and the PAIL OF WATER level.

OBJECT

To stretch the hamstrings of the raised leg, as well as the front of the thigh and the hip and ankle of the standing leg; also, to stretch the back as you lean over the leg.

STANCE CHECK

We are beginning to move your body into positions that vary greatly from the Stance. The challenge is for you to maintain the Stance—its alignment of parts relative to each other— as you move into these new positions. Here, the only variation from the Stance is in the legs. Can you maintain correct alignment from your hips to your head while assuming this new position of your legs? And can you keep your legs correct, with the knee under the hip and over the flexed ankle, even though your feet are turned out?

Now run through the Stance, standing on only one leg; this leg should be straighter than usual. Be aware of where you may feel you've moved off the alignment of the Stance.

Repeat on the other side.

NOTICE

How does each correction you may need to make to resume the Stance affect the stretch in your legs? As you become more correctly aligned, you'll be stretching further in the places where you're tight. Where you feel resistance is where you'll eventually feel and see change as you gradually release the places that are too contracted and tight, resulting in improper alignment. The pull of too-tight muscles will ease bit by bit as these muscles lengthen through stretching, allowing you to stand in this position with ease.

IF THIS IS IMPOSSIBLE

Try using a very low surface at first, such as a footstool or the seat of a couch. Don't worry if you can't straighten both legs at once, or even one at a time. Just work patiently at getting your legs up and out to some degree. Then drop the hip of the raised leg so that the PAIL OF WATER is level, straightening your legs when you've released further.

IF THIS IS EASY

Dropping your hip, tighten both thighs by contracting the muscles around your knees. Feel the extra challenge. Flex the foot of the raised leg, pressing the heel forward.

ADVANCED VERSION

Raise your arms up overhead and turn your torso toward the raised leg. Stretch your arms and head out and over, letting gravity pull you gently down and over the outstretched leg. Be aware of the increased stretch up the backs of your legs. What are you feeling in the outstretched leg? How about the groin? If you feel any discomfort there, back off a little and exhale *into* the painful place.

Eventually you'll be able to stretch your whole torso out and over, extending it along the outstretched leg. But be careful not to force it—*let* the hip and leg release, and *allow* the torso to move down toward the leg a little, to the point where you feel resistance. Pause, breathe into the area, let the hip and leg release, and let the torso move down a little farther.

Flex the foot of the raised leg for more stretch along the hamstrings.

14

WRISTS ON RAILING

Stretches arms, shoulders, back and legs

POSITION

Assume the Stance, facing the same railing or surface as in the previous movement but with your feet well back from it. Now bend at the hips and reach your arms out to place your wrists flat on the railing or surface. Walk your feet back until your arms and torso are at right angles to your legs. Bend your knees and keep your back flat. Extend your arms, locking the elbows. Keep your shoulders back and down. Let your head hang down, lengthening your neck. Feel the pull on your arms and upper back. Exhale. Rest, and repeat.

OBJECT

To stretch the arms, back and legs by forming a right angle. Imagine a straight line running up from your heels through your hips, and another, horizontal line running through your hips to your armpits to your elbows to your wrists and out the ends of your fingers. The railing or surface is providing the support to allow you really to stretch. You are hinged at ankles, knees and hips.

NOTICE

Does your back respond to the demand of this stretch by rounding and shortening? This is a common Creative Cheat for this position—the places that must be opened to permit this stretch are usually very tight, hence the temptation to "cheat creatively" and avoid the pain.

IF THIS IS IMPOSSIBLE

Bend your knees as deeply as you can. Drop one arm, letting it hang down to rest on your leg. Place the other wrist as far out to the side as necessary for you to drop that shoulder and lock the elbow. Now relax, dropping your head and feeling the release in your shoulder and back. Switch arms. Eventually you'll be able to stretch both arms out at once.

Flatten your back to send the stretch to your shoulders, then release your shoulders to stretch your arms and back.

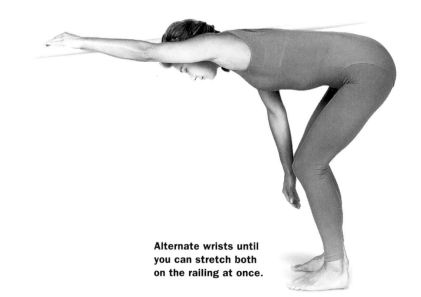

Alternate wrists until you can stretch both on the railing at once.

STANCE CHECK

Since this position involves a ninety-degree bend at the hips, how can you still maintain the coordinates of the Stance? Make sure the handle of the PLUNGER is sticking straight out ahead of you. (Here, "straight ahead" means pointing straight down at the floor.) Check your HEADLIGHTS and the ELASTIC BAND around your ankles. Keep the pressure outward on your knees (to maintain the tension in the ELASTIC BAND), even in this bent-over position. Keep inserting the SHIMS, lengthening the torso and sending the stretch into the shoulders.

IF THIS IS EASY

Make sure your back is flat, like a table with a tray on it. Straighten your bent knees as much as you can (without letting your calves go behind the line of gravity), while maintaining the flatness of your back.

ADVANCED VERSION

The basic position, except that your elbows are bent and your weight is resting on the upper arm near the elbow of the bent arm. Your head hangs between your elbows, and your hands are clasped over your head. Try to move your elbows closer together, relaxing your shoulders and neck.

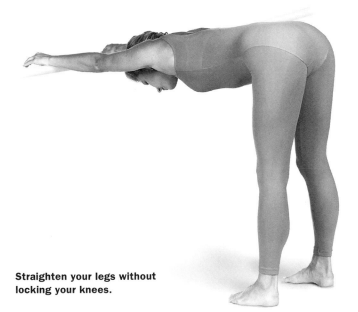

Straighten your legs without locking your knees.

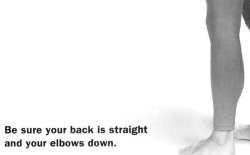

Be sure your back is straight and your elbows down.

115

STAIR CLIMB, UP AND DOWN (I)

15

Practices maintaining the Stance in a common activity; increases flexibility in ankle, knee and hip joints; strengthens thighs

UP THE STAIRS

POSITION

Stand at the bottom of a flight of stairs—the longer, the better. Supporting yourself by holding on to the banister, the wall, or both, place one foot flat on the first step, the heel resting on the step. (Your foot may turn slightly out to accommodate a small step; be sure to turn your knee and hip out as well, to stay aligned.) Let the ankle joint bend fully as you transfer your weight onto this leg. Bring the other leg through, and continue up the stairs.

Don't let your upper body tilt forward or back. Bend only at the ankles, knees and hips.

OBJECT

To rise higher in space while keeping your body aligned vertically, bending at ankle, knee and hip.

NOTICE

Watch to see if you bend anywhere other than at the hip, knee and ankle joints, as in the middle of the back or in the neck. Do you rise up on the balls of your feet, locking your knees, instead of keeping your heels down and your knees bent? Do you throw a hip out and a knee in as you change steps? Do you heave yourself from one step to the next?

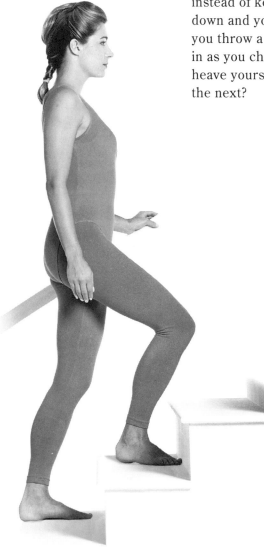

IF THIS IS IMPOSSIBLE

The ankle's flexibility is crucial to the opening of the joints above it. Practice #5 (Heel Drop on Stairs) until the ankle joint and Achilles tendon release and lengthen further. As you do Up the Stairs, make sure you're holding on very securely with your hand. (Your brain will not let you try something as scary as walking unless you have support.) Think the Stance and feel yourself walking into it, reestablishing it, at each step. Go ahead and *pull* yourself up if you must at first so that you don't bend inappropriately in a Creative Cheat. Then gradually relax the help as your legs become more flexible and stronger.

IF THIS IS EASY

Try to make the transition smooth from one leg to the other, with no hitch as you shift legs. Bend more deeply at the ankle, knee and hip to get more stretch in the muscles and a stronger workout in the legs, especially in the thighs. Make sure you open the RACCOON EYES fully, smoothing the fronts of your thighs and your abdomen, and keep the PAIL OF WATER level.

THE IMPORTANCE OF GOING UP AND DOWN STAIRS PROPERLY

Climbing up and down stairs is an easy way to develop and reinforce good habits of alignment. It's also one of the easiest activities to do incorrectly.

A classic example of a Creative Cheat is the way most people climb stairs, which readily lends itself to an alternate way of covering the distance when the joints and muscles that should be doing the work are too stiff and short and weak to function properly. To see how you might be compensating, watch other people as they go up and down stairs. See how far they fall out of the Stance (even farther, usually, than when walking.) Are they hunched over, rounding the back and pulling themselves up by the banister? Do they throw one hip out to the side as they descend? Or do they bounce down, using momentum to get over the tight spots? Each Creative Cheat, in its attempt to circumvent using a tight or shortened place in the body, avoids pressing through the joint to keep it open and released.

Walk up and down stairs yourself as slowly as possible, noticing where and how the Stance may be difficult to maintain. Does the handle of the PLUNGER dip as you go up? Do the HEADLIGHTS turn out, or do your knee joints lock? Does the PAIL OF WATER tip forward or to one side? The more gracefully you can go up and down, the more efficiently you'll be working the muscles that help to move you effortlessly while you maintain the Stance.

117

15

STAIR CLIMB, UP AND DOWN (II)

Practices maintaining the Stance in a common activity; increases flexibility in ankle, knee and hip joints; strengthens thighs

DOWN THE STAIRS

POSITION

From the top step, extend one foot and point the toes. Step down on the toes first, then roll back along the foot, through the arch, to land on the heel. As the heel makes contact, immediately bend the ankle and knee joints, pressing squarely on the foot. Feel the muscles of the thigh working, and keep the PAIL OF WATER level. How much outward pressure must you exert on your thighs to keep your knees from dropping inward? Probably more than you think, especially if your feet and ankles are tight and you have knee problems.

OBJECT

To sink lower in space by hinging at the joints, keeping the torso erect as you "slink" down the stairs.

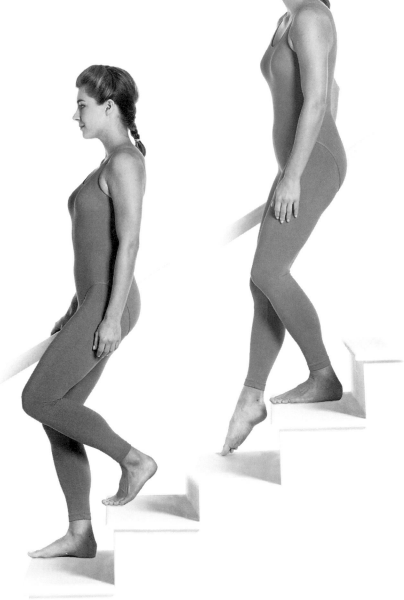

When going up or down stairs, keep your movements smooth and the ankle, knee and hip joints flexed. Point your toes strongly when descending.

NOTICE

Do you want to lock the rear leg and almost fall forward, landing too heavily on the heel of the foot? Or do you bend forward at the hips to avoid bending the ankle?

IF THIS IS IMPOSSIBLE

Hold on tightly to the banister or wall. Point your toes more than you think necessary; imagine that your toes are the head of a snake as it starts to slither down. Press firmly on the back ankle while that foot is still on the step. Load up the front leg with weight. Hold the Stance, then bring the next leg through.

IF THIS IS EASY

Use this as a strengthening movement throughout the day. Feel how much good pressure you're asking your legs to take as you keep tall and aligned, allowing the hinges to really work.

PERFECT BALANCE

Balance is not something you either were or were not born with, like curly hair or blue eyes. It is simply the even, equal relationship of the muscles holding you up. It is an innate ability that can be uncovered with practice. Balance happens effortlessly as your muscles become flexible, strong and responsive, and as you begin to sense where you need to adjust your alignment to experience the still, centered point of gravity. Imagine a sailboat out on a lake and the surge in its sails as it finds the wind's path; in the same way, your body will lift up in gravity at just the place where there is no drag caused by misalignment.

When you're just beginning to do balancing movements, be confident that you will soon develop the muscles and correct placement you need for balance by acting as if you already had access to them. Knowing that balance does exist for you, and expecting suddenly to find yourself in it, will help you persist in the subtle search long enough for the body-mind to fill in the gap between intention and execution. You will in fact have what you thought you never had or what you've been pretending to have: perfect balance.

16

GROUCHO WALK

Increases flexibility of ankles and knees in walking; increases strength and stability of legs

POSITION

Assume the Stance. Take one step forward, and stop. Make sure you're still in the Stance, even though one leg is ahead of the other. Continue taking slow, deliberate steps, letting your weight sink down from your waist into the hip, knee and ankle joints with each step, while continuing to rise tall in the torso.

OBJECT

To exaggerate the bend of ankles and knees, and to keep them very bent throughout the entire movement; also, to inhibit the tendency to straighten the rear leg as you walk.

NOTICE

As you walk, do you feel that you want to *rise up* with each step rather than *sink down* as you should here? Be aware how difficult it is to resist rising up. Do you feel yourself leaning forward, bending at the waist in order to avoid bending at hip, knee and ankle? Do your knees fall in, rather than stay out in line with your hips and ankles?

IF THIS IS IMPOSSIBLE

Watching yourself in the mirror, hold on to a wall or railing. Take one step, being aware of what you must do to keep flexed in the joints. Imagine a mark at the top of your head that must be kept level; don't let your head bob up and down as you move from step to step. Just at the point where you want to go *up,* increase the

Set the heel of the forward foot down, then the arch, ball and toes in sequence.

Let your weight sink down from the waist into the hip, knee and ankle with each step, pressing the rear heel down as you move forward.

bend, hold on tighter, *use* your arms for support and begin to *trust* this leg. Press outward, keeping the letter "H" in place. Allow your legs to feel very weak; they'll get stronger after a while, but they must first *feel.*

IF THIS IS EASY

As you do the movement, pay close attention to the mechanics of your feet. Consciously set the heel of the forward foot down, then the arch, the ball and the toes, in sequence. At the same time, bend at the ankle and knee, and open the hip joint (the RACCOON EYE), pressing the hip slightly forward so that it's fully over the foot.

Keep pressing the rear heel into the floor, resisting your natural inclination to lift it. Once your weight is firmly on the forward leg, balance on that leg as you shift all the weight onto it and swing the rear leg through to begin the sequence again. *Walking is sequential balancing.*

Pay special attention to the position of the pelvis and the PAIL OF WATER. It is the unconscious tilting forward of the pelvis, because of shortened Achilles tendons, hamstrings and hip flexor muscles, that tilts the small of the back forward and

tightens it, causing back pain. *Press firmly down on the rear leg as you go forward for the additional support you need to keep the pelvis level. This will also make it possible for your abdominal muscles to work together with your back muscles.*

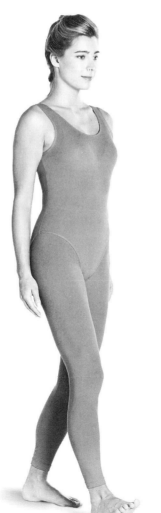

Keep the hip, knee and ankle joints flexed.

ADVANCED VERSION

After you can do several laps around the house, loping like Groucho Marx, modify the walk to a more normal one. Gradually decrease the extreme bend in your knees, while maintaining the deep bend in your ankles and opening the RACCOON EYES. Notice the expanded role of your feet and ankles as you walk. You're now using them much more actively, to their fullest capacity as hinges.

THE IMPORTANCE OF LENGTH IN WALKING

In your old way of standing, with locked knees, your legs tightened and shortened along the back. Every time you took a step, instead of letting the joints bend fully, you locked at a certain point in the movement and stuck there, forced to resort to a Creative Cheat to compensate for the loss of length in the leg owing to insufficient flexing at the joints. You had to rise up with each step since sinking down was closed to you, blocked by the tightness. This is frequently the cause of discomfort in the lower back. The energy that should be moving freely down and up from the waist is locked in, compressing the spine and causing pain.

When the muscles in your legs have begun to lengthen and release as you practice the Groucho Walk and other movements, you'll soon be able to sink deeply down on your front leg, with a strong bend in the ankle and an Achilles tendon long enough to permit this deep bend. This allows your spine to be brought forward in space so that it is no longer compressed but lifted by gravity.

THE VANCE STANCE

Develops leg muscles for power and balance

POSITION

Kneeling on the floor, extend one leg forward to a ninety-degree angle and place the sole of the foot flat, ready to take your weight. Flex the toes of the other foot and use them to help push you up. Lift your torso upright, with the handle of the PLUNGER aiming straight out in front of you (not toward the floor). Let your arms swing forward as if you were reaching for a life raft.

OBJECT

To form a right angle with the forward leg, and to push off with the rear foot and toes so that you stand up using mostly the leg muscles (not the muscles of the back), with no bracing from the arms and hands.

NOTICE

Do you tend to bend at the waist as you try to get up? Does your knee fall inward? Is your impulse to push off with some part of your arm or hand? These are all Creative Cheats, deflecting you from developing strength in weaker muscles. Resist the impulse to go with the old, easier way; persevere in the new.

The foot of the forward leg must be far enough from your body to allow the knee to bend. As you swing your arms forward, push your torso up with the help of your toes.

Reach out farther with your hands as you begin to rise.

IF THIS IS IMPOSSIBLE

Hold on to a stable piece of furniture and align yourself correctly. Use plenty of arm muscle to make up for weak thigh muscles. Be aware of exactly which muscles are being asked to do the work, and gradually allow more and more weight on your legs.

Check to see if the foot of your forward leg is too close to your body; *it must be far enough in*

Use a stationary object for support, allowing more and more weight on your legs, until you're able to do this movement with ease.

front to allow your knee to bend well forward without forcing your foot up onto the toes. The ankle joint should hinge; don't let your foot roll up onto your toes. Probably you need to move the foot a little farther forward. Be sure to press down firmly with the heel. This may make it more difficult at first, but eventually the movement will become easier if you engage the heel and make the thigh begin to work.

IF THIS IS EASY

Be sure to keep your back erect. Rise up as slowly and smoothly as possible, hinging well at the hip joints. This movement will help develop control and strength in your thighs and feet.

ADVANCED VERSION

From the Stance, place one foot behind and reverse the movement: lower yourself slowly to kneeling, arms out to the side as if you were balancing on a tightrope. Feel the delicate balance between your feet and the muscles being used in your thighs and hips.

THE IMPORTANCE OF GETTING UP AND DOWN PROPERLY

Part of our work involves instilling painless new habits to reinforce the new access to unfamiliar muscles, so that you learn instinctively to use the correct ones—and only those. We will be practicing the movements and activities of everyday life and learning how to carry them out with awareness, always maintaining the Stance.

Observe people at a party or lecture who are seated on the floor; notice how they struggle to their feet, holding on to something stable and then pulling themselves up, or bracing a forearm against a knee and pressing themselves up. They are using the strength of their *arms* or their *skeletal system*, not the leg muscles, and neither way allows or encourages reliance on elastic muscle strength. Either way is a Creative Cheat. If you suspect that you don't have the strength required to stand, you use your body weight against the object or the bent knee. You can "stand" this way, but you have avoided the use of your leg muscles that keep you strong and youthful. Since you *can* "stand" this way, you think you *should*. However, the end result is a gradual deterioration and weakening of your legs. The downward spiral continues: the less you *use* your legs, the less you *can* use them.

Happily, the more you deepen your awareness of the most efficient way of moving, the more fully you will develop the many subtle and specialized muscles you have at your disposal, enabling you to avoid overusing some muscles at the expense of others. (This, incidentally, is one of the most important secrets of aging gracefully.)

18

ANKLE SIT

Stretches muscles along front of foot and ankle while contracting Achilles tendon and hamstrings; eventually opens thigh muscles

POSITION

Sit on the floor Japanese style, on your knees with your buttocks down on your heels and the tops of your feet against the floor. (If this is too difficult, add large pillows between the backs of your thighs and your lower legs.) Your knees are slightly apart, with your big toes just touching, and your heels drop slightly away from each other, to the outside. Try to stretch the entire foot and shin area with the rest of your body sitting back and down against your lower legs.

This is a very important position to practice, especially if you have foot problems. The ankle and foot need to be both stretched and contracted (released and strengthened) to provide you with a strong, flexible base. We have already stretched the Achilles tendon and contracted the front of the foot in #5 (Heel Drop on Stairs). Now we will reverse the stretch, flattening and stretching the front while contracting the Achilles tendon.

When you're able to rest your weight back fully on your lower legs, you'll feel additional pressure all the way through the arch of your foot and out the toes, lengthening the muscles of the top of the foot. This is what we want, the sense of "pressing out" tight spots in the body, here in a part of the foot that is seldom stretched. When this is open, you'll be able to allow the stretch into the thighs, so necessary for becoming strong.

OBJECT

To use all your resting body weight to stretch the front of the lower leg and foot while contracting the Achilles tendon and the hamstrings in the back of the leg, folding the body by hinging at the knee and hip.

NOTICE

Are your ankles always held fixed in a right angle, seemingly "frozen," unable to stretch? This is not uncommon, especially in people with foot and back problems. The alignment of your entire body will improve when you can get the front of the ankle joint flat on the floor, so persevere.

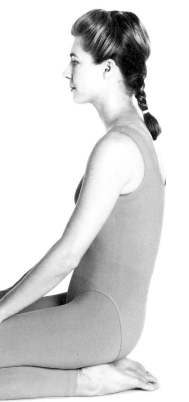

With knees slightly apart and big toes touching, rest your weight on your lower legs.

IF THIS IS IMPOSSIBLE

Don't despair; this may well be the most difficult movement in the entire series for you even to attempt if you're stiff in the ankle joints—and that's where most people are tightest. Rigid ankle joints are among the most common of "frozennesses," because it's *possible* to get about without articulating the ankle joint, moving only at knee and hip. (Often people whose bodies are very tight are convinced that the human body is not meant to open this way: they think it is as if we were asking the *elbow* joint to reverse! Not so. Your ankles *will* open, eventually, and you will understand their importance.)

Put a rolled-up thick quilt or sleeping bag, or a pile of pillows, in the fold of your legs between the back of the thighs and the calves. Get as much height as you need to begin actually to sit with reasonable comfort. As you approach being able to let your full weight rest on your heels, gradually decrease the amount of padding until you're sitting with your bottom resting right on your feet. (This can be a slow, sometimes painful area to open. Know that the more it hurts, the more crucial it is to open here.)

IF THIS IS EASY

If you can immediately sit flat on your ankles, rejoice—you have very free, open, flexible feet.

ADVANCED VERSION

From the sitting position, slouch down (to send the stretch into your thighs and to protect your back), place your hands on the floor behind you with your fingers pointing forward, tuck your pelvis under and roll gently back onto your ankles, all the way to your toes, so that they take even more of your weight. Your knees have lifted off the floor, and you're sitting with your back at about a forty-five degree angle to the floor. Come back to sitting squarely on your ankles, and release.

Place a pillow in the fold of your legs until your ankle joints lose their rigidity.

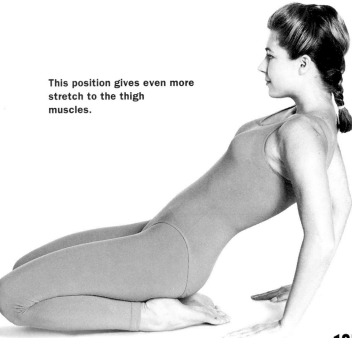

This position gives even more stretch to the thigh muscles.

19

TOE BEND, ACHILLES STRETCH

Stretches Achilles tendons, arches and undersides of toes

POSITION

From the basic position of #18 (sitting flat on your ankles, with or without padding), lean forward with your weight on your hands. Lift your knees up and turn your toes under, flexing to a right angle at the toe joints, and lift the heels up, keeping your legs and feet together so they touch at the inner ankle bones. Now, with your knees still lifted, press *back* onto your heels, feeling the pull on the Achilles tendons as you press your heels down strongly toward the floor, still with your toes hinged. Begin to lower your knees back to the floor as you simultaneously press your heels down strongly the other way, creating a stretch all along your calves as well as down the Achilles tendons.

OBJECT

To stretch the Achilles tendons in a new way; to stretch the arches; to bend the toes (especially the big toe).

NOTICE

Are you able to bend your big toes enough so that you can lift your heels to form right angles? If so, get your heels to move toward the floor in this position. Also, check to see if your heels are moving apart rather than staying together, ankle bones meeting.

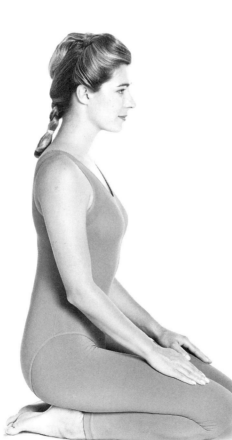

Begin in the Ankle Sit position.

From the Ankle Sit, lean forward with your weight on your hands. Flex your ankles and form right angles with your toes, lifting your knees.

IF THIS IS IMPOSSIBLE

Squat down with your feet flat on the floor. Using your arms for support, try to bring your feet together. Now gently press your heels down, without trying to raise them first to bend your toes. If your problem is hinging the toes, do #9 (Toe Crunch Series) to open the joint. Eventually, by contracting the Achilles tendons, you can raise your heels, then begin to drop them.

IF THIS IS EASY

While slowly pressing your knees to touch the floor, direct the stretch down the Achilles tendons with as much pressure as you can manage. Feel how your arches and feet open up from this two-way stretch down the calves and Achilles tendons.

Keeping your legs and feet together, press your knees forward as you press your heels back toward the floor.

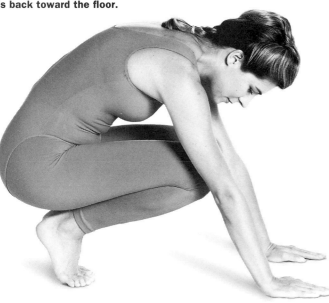

"HE'S WALKING LIKE AN OLD MAN!"

CONRAD'S STORY

Several years ago a lively, attractive woman in her mid-eighties was referred to me for help with a nagging hip problem. She made rapid progress after we uncovered a broken ankle from thirty years before, the source of a longstanding compensation that caused her almost to limp as she walked. We established a new pattern of alignment that not only relieved the pain in her hip but gave her a whole new sense of ease and confidence in everything she did.

Pleased with her progress, she brought her neighbor to one of our sessions. They had been sweethearts for many years—he was ninety-two at the time I met him. "You must do something for him," she said. "He's starting to walk like an old man!" And sure enough, watching him in his first session, we all noticed that he walked with a stooped, shuffling gait, sliding his feet along. He *did* look like an old man—a caricature of one. It turned out that his ankles and shins were painfully frozen from way back and had grown even tighter as his fear of falling and breaking a hip had become greater. And this increasing immobility made him still more insecure on his feet, so that he locked even tighter. His whole body was affected by this stiffness in his lower body.

Gradually, Conrad learned how to bend at his ankles and knees deeply enough to engage his thigh muscles. Day by day, he saw and felt himself improving. Now, when he climbed stairs, he could use his leg muscles instead of pulling himself up with his arms and back, which involved muscles not designed for this purpose and caused his hunched-over gait. "I'm more flexible now than I was at seventy-five, seventeen years ago," he told me. "I know how to let my *legs* do the work—they're getting stronger all the time as I use them more. And I can protect my back and keep it tall and long."

20

CROSS-LEGGED SIT

Opens hip joints, knees and ankles; releases all along sides of legs and buttocks

POSITION

Sit on the floor with your legs crossed in front of you, not tucked under each other but positioned so that one is in front of the other on the floor. Make fists behind your back and push up from your knuckles, keeping your elbows locked to form a rigid brace to support your torso as you sit tall. Point your toes and lay your legs flat. Feel the stretch especially in the outside of the hip of the forward leg. Reverse legs, and rest. Repeat.

OBJECT

To rest the entire leg flat on the floor, with the side of the knee against the floor, and at the same time to sit straight and tall, with no support.

NOTICE

Do your knees and legs rise off the floor? Does your back want to slouch? Do you feel a painful pull in your knees, especially the one in front? These are all signs that you need *more length*. Think of releasing more deeply in the hips—mentally direct the flow of energy out of your hips into your knees and out along your toes. At the same time, imagine the *sap* rising up, lifting your torso tall and straight. Each command helps the other.

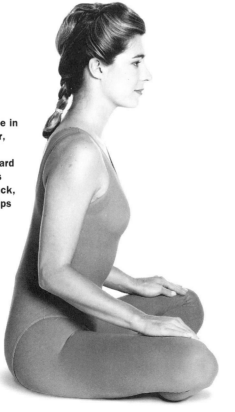

One leg should be in front of the other, not overlapping. Pressing down hard on your knuckles helps lift your back, which in turn helps lower your legs.

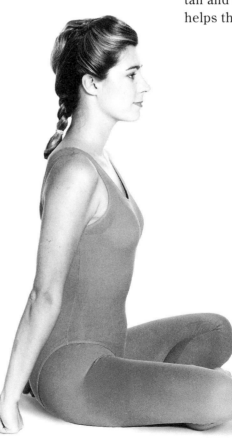

When your back muscles become stronger, place your hands in your lap.

STANCE CHECK

In this seated position, where does your PLUNGER handle point? What has happened to your PAIL OF WATER? (Both the PLUNGER handle and the PAIL OF WATER should be level, parallel to the floor.) What's happening to the ACCORDION at the back of your neck? (It should be expanded, your neck long.) Is your head level, with your eyes level and straight ahead? Are you able to create space in your midsection for the SHIMS to be inserted so that your torso can lengthen?

Feel how pressing down hard on your knuckles helps to lift your back, which in turn helps to lower your legs. Feel how pointing your feet strongly helps your back to lift. *(Remember the two-way flow of energy.)*

IF THIS IS IMPOSSIBLE

Ask a friend to sit on the floor behind you, leaning back on his or her hands, feet pressing against the middle of your back. See how this added support helps you to sit taller, creating *more length* all the way up. This frees the hips to drop down and the spine to move forward. Gradually transfer the work of your friend's feet to your own arms, propping yourself up with both hands as the feet are removed. (Instead of a friend, you can use the edge of the seat of a chair whose back is against a wall, for stability and support, and a throw pillow to increase the angle just a bit.) Remember to continue relaxing in the hips, thinking (directing) the energy to flow out into the knees. Then gradually take one hand off the floor and feel what happens. Feel how *you* must hold yourself up from within. Feel a new use of your back. When you can, remove the other hand, too.

IF THIS IS EASY

Sit tall with your hands in your lap, palms up. Gently drop your head forward, letting your neck gradually release into length. Feel the stretch all up and down your spine.

21

CROSS-LEGGED SIT: HEAD TO FLOOR

Opens hip joints (a more intense stretch than #20); lengthens muscles of neck and back

POSITION

From the basic position of #20, gently drop your head forward, feeling the stretch all the way down your spine. Let your head drop all the way to the floor, if possible, paying special attention to the back of your neck. This is the key area to be released, giving you the experience of feeling how much tightness is stored there. Let your head dangle freely, like a wilting flower.

Place your palms and elbows flat on the floor in front of you and continue rolling down until your head touches the floor. Reverse legs. Repeat.

OBJECT

To use the position of the body and the weight of the head to let the spine lengthen and round as fully as possible. Remember to *let* your head drop toward the floor; don't *push* it down. Stay with the *process* of the slow, gradual lengthening of the neck and spine; don't rush toward the end result of touching your head to the floor. It's unimportant if your head gets all the way down to the floor. The purpose of this movement is to experience the process of lengthening, moment to moment, without concern for what the final position will be.

NOTICE

Do your buttocks rise up off the floor as you lean over? If so, stop leaning; pause until your hips and back have released further. Now drop your head again, releasing your neck a little further. Place your hands on the floor in front of you and push your weight back, then continue.

If you feel an ache deep in the hinge of the knee, usually of the forward leg, most probably

Begin in the cross-legged position, one leg in front of the other.

Roll down slowly, keeping your buttocks on the floor; let your head drop down, gradually stretching your neck and spine until your hips and back release to allow your head to touch the floor.

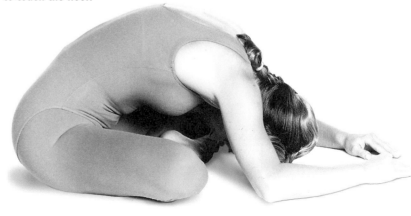

you're feeling the effects of bowlegs or knock-knees. It's likely that your knee joint has not been correctly hinged in a long time. The normal resting angle for the knee joints of bowlegs or knock-knees is not this acute (narrow). And now you are, in a sense, coming up against the limits imposed by your old tightness. Pointing your toes more strongly should help ease the pain. (This is both a "good" pain and a "bad" pain: it's signaling you to make an adjustment or you'll hurt yourself, but it's not sending you a message to stop altogether.)

IF THIS IS IMPOSSIBLE

Just let your head hang down, feeling the strong stretch along the back of your neck, staying with it and breathing into your neck as it releases. Notice what happens as you think of exhaling into the point of most discomfort. Continue pointing your feet and toes, allowing your knee joints to release. (If the knee pain is deep in the hinge of the joint, put a pillow under each knee until the "rust" of old misalignment is eliminated.) At the same time, concentrate on releasing in the hip and back, with the energy that is freed by the release flowing down out of the hip into the knee and out the foot and toes.

IF THIS IS EASY

When your head can rest easily on the floor, lift your chin and aim it farther out, as if to push it along the floor. Then drop your head down again, noticing how much closer to the floor your torso now is. Also note how you've brought more tight places into your awareness. Breathe into these places, as you think of releasing them *on* the breath.

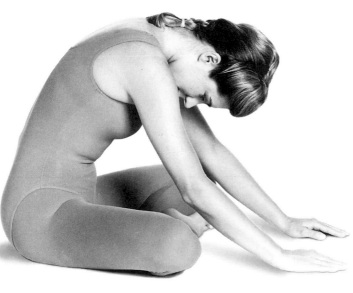

If touching your head to the floor is too difficult, just drop your head to release your neck and spine; be sure to keep your buttocks and thighs on the floor.

CROSS-LEGGED SIT: ELBOWS UP AND OUT

Increases flexibility and mobility in shoulders; flattens "dowager's hump"

POSITION

From the basic position of #20, sit up tall with your legs crossed on the floor. Drop your shoulders so that they rest easily in the MILKMAID'S YOKE, and place your hands on your shoulders, fingers pointing back. Bring your elbows together; now lift your elbows up and over your head, keeping them as close together as possible until they have to separate: rotate your arms out to the side, back and down. Do several circles.

OBJECT

To rotate the shoulders, using the arms as levers; also, to maintain a tall, strong back while the arms move independently and to teach the upper back to contract properly.

NOTICE

How tight are your shoulder joints? It may be difficult to move your shoulders and arms separately from your back and neck (or, indeed, from the rest of your body). Are you hunching your shoulders?

Sitting upright, bring your elbows together in front.

Keeping your spine tall, raise your elbows until you have to separate them.

Drop your shoulders, pulling the shoulder blades together.

IF THIS IS IMPOSSIBLE

Get a friend to press your back straight with his or her knee from behind and grasp your elbows to raise them up overhead, pull them out to the side, then rotate them all around and down. Drop your shoulders forcibly from within as your arms are moved.

IF THIS IS EASY

Watch yourself in the mirror; make sure that your shoulders stay down the entire time.

ADVANCED VERSION

From the middle of the movement, when your elbows are extended out to the side (before coming down), contract your shoulder blades together and turn your hands out to the sides with the palms down, Egyptian style. Keep your hands in this position as you release your shoulder blades; pinch them together again, and place your hands in your lap, palms up.

See and feel where your shoulders belong. Now release the grip, trying to keep your shoulders in the same position, without the necessity of pulling your shoulder blades together.

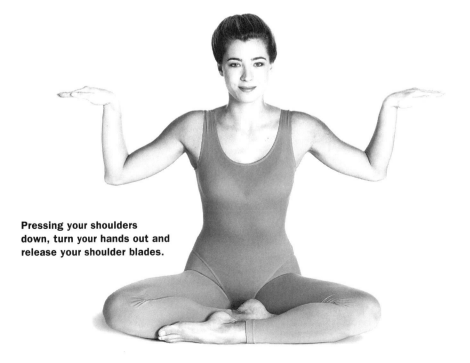

Pressing your shoulders down, turn your hands out and release your shoulder blades.

THE VANCE STANCE

Stretches
hamstrings
and back

POSITION

From the basic position of #20, extend one leg out straight in front of you, angled a little out to the side, ankle flexed. Lift your arms overhead, clasping your thumbs, and bend at the hip joint (not at the waist) to stretch your arms out along the outstretched leg. Keep your buttocks and the outer thigh of the bent leg on the floor as you twist from the waist toward the outstretched leg. Gradually lower your head to touch the leg. Exhale, releasing still further down toward the leg as your breath moves out.

Reverse. Repeat.

OBJECT

To stretch the outstretched leg and the back.

Be sure your PAIL OF WATER is level from side to side and front to back as you lift your arms overhead.

NOTICE

Is tightness along the back of your outstretched leg interfering with flexing at your hip? Do you feel tightness in your back or, farther up, in your neck and shoulder area? Notice whether there is a difference in your legs: is the tighter leg on the side where you're tight in other places? There *is* a connection!

IF THIS IS IMPOSSIBLE

Perhaps you're not hinging properly at the hip joint. Prop yourself up on your knuckles, concentrating on sitting tall, with your PAIL OF WATER level from side to side as well as from front to back. Feel your entire back working as a unit, from the bottom of your buttocks to the top of your head, so that you don't collapse in the middle. Then drop your head forward and just wait there, exhaling with awareness into the tight places. Let your hands rest on your thigh or ankle.

IF THIS IS EASY

Release for *still more length* in your back and legs. Lock your fingers under your calf by really extending your leg; drop your head forward and use the strength of your arms to pull your torso and head gently toward your leg. Then place your arms alongside your leg, elbows flat, hands around your foot.

Lift yourself up out of your hips and twist to the side before you bend over.

Keep your buttocks on the floor as you use the strength of your arms to pull your torso and head forward over your extended leg.

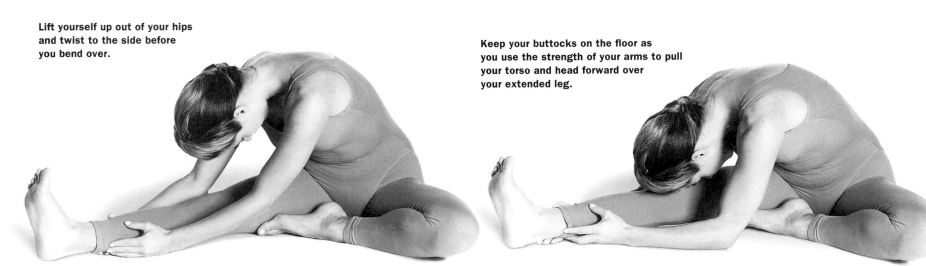

24

SITTING FORWARD BEND

Stretches hamstrings and back (a more intense stretch than #23)

POSITION

Sit upright with your legs extended in front of you, ankles flexed. Lean your torso out over your legs as far as possible, hands resting on legs, neck relaxed and head down.

OBJECT

Ultimately, to extend the whole length of the torso flat out along the legs, with the elbows resting on the floor alongside. It is essential to keep the legs straight, with thighs locked.

NOTICE

Is this difficult? Don't worry—with patience you'll get there. This is one of the tightest lines in the body. The temptation is to try to get your head down onto your knees at once. Instead, stay with the *process* of gradually lengthening the hamstrings and the muscles all along your back, especially the lower back and neck. Go slowly and breathe into the tightness, wherever you feel it. This is truly the fastest way to change.

You may want to begin this movement with your arms lifted overhead. Be sure your torso is lifted up from your hips and that the SHIMS are in place.

As you stretch out your hamstrings and back, you'll be able to rest the entire length of your torso along your legs.

136

IF THIS IS IMPOSSIBLE

Simply drop your head down toward your chest and stop at the first point that hurts. Stay with it, and feel the rush of release down the length of your spine. This is often quite intense, but the tightness *must* be released for a healthy, pain-free back. (The paradox is that in order to eradicate the "bad" pain from your back, you must go through and release the "good" pain.) When you're able to focus on the exact location of the pain, you're

making progress. At whatever point you can stay with your head hanging down comfortably, stop and breathe into it. Continue a little farther, then stop when it begins to hurt and breathe into it. Stay there awhile.

As you relax into these places, you may feel pain all up and down your spine and legs. Your feet may also go to sleep. This is normal, but if you're too uncomfortable at any given point, back off. There will be a place where you can just "hang out" easily; that will be your starting point.

Don't forget to breathe. Breathing into the tight and painful places should be an integral part of this stretch (and of all the other stretches; the difference is that here the breathing is even more intimately linked with your ability to do the stretch at all). And remember: you will progress much more quickly by *going slowly* into the stretch and releasing from within on the breath rather than by *forcing* it.

IF THIS IS EASY

Lift your head as if to extend both your chin and your ribs out over your knees. This will create *more length* at the hips by exerting a greater pull on the hamstrings. When you're extended out as far as you can go, lower your head and feel the increased stretch. As this becomes easy, add a still stronger pull by lacing your hands around your feet, elbows on the floor.

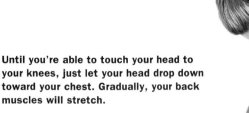

Until you're able to touch your head to your knees, just let your head drop down toward your chest. Gradually, your back muscles will stretch.

Stretches spine;
opens hip
flexors

POSITION

Lying on your back, pull your knees against your chest with both hands, lengthening the back of your neck as you do so. Resist the impulse to compress and shorten your back—keep lengthening all the way up as you pull your knees in. Keep the back of your neck long and your head flat on the floor. You should be facing the ceiling—don't let your head tilt back. Try to get the tops of your thighs flat against your chest, with the insides touching each other.

OBJECT

To stretch the spine from the tail-bone to the back of the neck, by applying pressure on the legs, and to open the hip flexors (the RACCOON EYES) by contracting them.

NOTICE

Locate any resistance in your hip joints (the RACCOON EYES) and *breathe into it*; that is, pretend that your breath is moving into the hips as you inhale, and moving out through the legs and back as you exhale, releasing the tension there.

Feel what happens in the small of your back. Does it tilt forward and shorten? And your neck—does it shorten, tipping your head back? What can you do to keep your neck *as flat as possible,* in contact with the floor almost all the way up? As always, the answer is to think *more length.*

Keep the small of your back flat on the floor as you pull on your knees and try to get the tops of your thighs to rest flat against your chest.

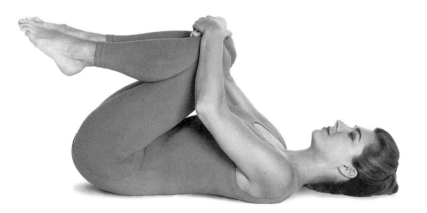

IF THIS IS IMPOSSIBLE

If you have difficulty keeping your head flat on the floor, or if it tends to tilt back or not to touch the floor at all, put a pillow beneath it. Place one foot on the floor, knee bent. Press back to flatten the small of your back. As you apply pressure with your hands, pull on just one knee at a time. Go easy until you can keep your neck long at the same time as you press your knee to your chest. If you feel your neck shortening in response to the pressure of your hands, stop, rethink length in your neck, then try to press a little further. This hip joint is often very tight and painful to release, especially if you have swayback or scoliosis. Persist, for this is the gateway to your back. Then try it with two legs, but let the legs fall wide apart at first. Gradually try to bring them closer as the hips open.

IF THIS IS EASY

Lift your head up to touch your forehead first to one knee, then to the other. Lengthen the back of your neck as you lower your head back down to the floor. Be sure to exhale as you touch your forehead to your knees, and press your shoulders back and down.

ADVANCED VERSION

Touch your head to both knees, then let go with your hands, continuing to touch your head to your knees. Exhale. Shoulders back and down.

Keep your back flat and your neck long as you pull your knee in.

Alternate legs as you bring your knee to your forehead. Once the movement is comfortable, let your hands go while you continue to touch your head to your knees.

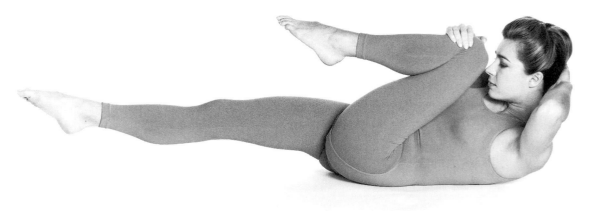

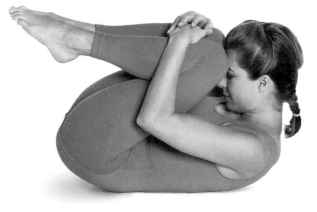

26

DEAD BUG

Opens hip joints; stretches groin and spine

POSITION

Lying flat on your back, legs in the air with knees bent, reach between your legs and grasp your heels. Open your legs as wide as you can, keeping a right angle at the hip joints and your feet flexed, soles toward the ceiling.

Let one knee drop over toward the outside to touch the floor, maintaining the wide angle of your legs with your hands holding your heels. Come back up to center, then drop the same knee over to the other side to touch the floor. Repeat, exhaling as the knee drops toward the floor.

OBJECT

To keep the hip joints flexed, forming right angles between the back and hips, and between the feet and ankles, while pressing the knees open; also, to drop the knees over to one side, one at a time, in order to release in the hip joints.

NOTICE

Feel the interconnectedness of your hips, feet and neck. Do you find that you shorten your neck in order to reach your feet, and that you have trouble contracting in the hip joints? Is it painful to open the groin while your hands hold on to your feet? As you tilt over to one side to touch your knee to the floor, can you keep your neck long and your hips released and open? Do your legs want to pull away from your body to block the release of tension in your hips?

Cup your heels with your hands, keeping your legs as open and wide as you can.

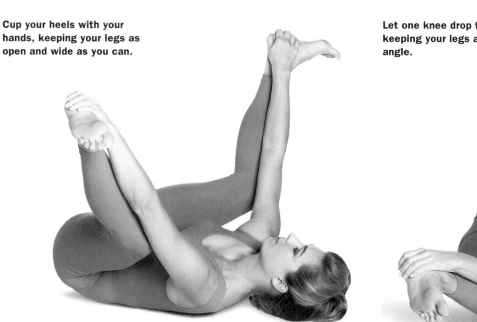

Let one knee drop to the floor, keeping your legs at a wide angle.

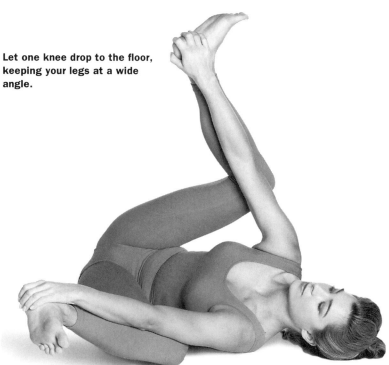

IF THIS IS IMPOSSIBLE

Work on just getting your back flat and your neck long on the floor with your knees over your chest; don't pull on them. When you can do this, gently grasp your ankles. Notice whatever discomfort you may feel—it will usually be in the hip joints or the groin. Breathe into the discomfort. Then just let your knees drop out a little, then return to the starting position; don't worry if at first you don't actually touch one knee to the floor. Letting your knees drop apart is an important first step. Concentrate on maintaining an open, stretched feeling between your legs. When this area is tight, it is usually *very* tight. Go gently.

IF THIS IS EASY

Lower each knee to the floor, one at a time. Work on releasing the hip joint so that only the leg moves to touch the knee to the floor, not any part of the upper body. Keep the top leg almost upright and stationary, letting the other leg drop independently. Keep your back still.

ADVANCED VERSION

With your knees open, legs wide and up in the air, and feet flexed, let go of your ankles and reach your arms, shoulders and head out between your legs, contracting the abdominals as you reach with the upper body. Reach through, with the hands and pulse forward and back, in very small movements, for a count of twenty. Release, and repeat.

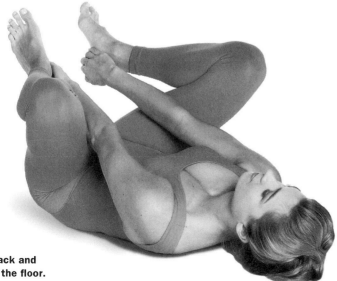

Keep your back and neck flat on the floor.

27

PELVIS FLATTEN AND ARCH

Releases and contracts lower back; increases mobility and strength of spine

POSITION

Lying flat on your back with your arms out to the side and palms up, draw your knees toward your chest so that the small of your back can flatten against the floor. Lower your feet until they're flat on the floor. Try to keep the small of your back flat by pressing against the floor with your feet and bent legs.

OBJECT

Alternately to arch and flatten the small of the back by first contracting the muscles of the lower back, then releasing them into length. (Think first of making a tunnel, arching your back to let a toy truck pass underneath you; then, after the truck goes through, lower your back as you press your waist into the floor.) Also, to engage the abdominals to work with the back, strengthening the torso and back.

NOTICE

Does the back of your neck feel connected to the small of your back at the other end of your spine? As you arch your back, feel your neck contract in response, giving away some of its length in order to allow you to arch. Now, as you flatten your back, feel the choice you have: to let your neck remain tight and shortened or, with an act of awareness, to *lengthen* it, consciously continuing to release it and stretch it in a line from your hairline to infinity as your back finally flattens.

Keep your back flat on the floor by contracting your abdominal muscles and pressing back through your legs. Next, arch your back. Then press your waist into the floor, lengthening your neck as you flatten the small of your back.

142

IF THIS IS IMPOSSIBLE

Try for whatever movement is possible; emphasize the arching. If flattening is very difficult, you probably have a deeply swayed back. Practice lying with your arms wrapped around one leg, while the foot of the other leg stays flat on the floor, knee bent. Pull your leg into your chest as you press the other foot against the floor to help tilt your pelvis back to get your back flat. Reverse legs.

IF THIS IS EASY

After you've done a few arches and releases, press the small of your back down flat and see how far you can walk your feet away, almost straightening your legs and still keeping your back flat. Be aware of what this new pressure feels like, especially as it affects the tops of your thighs in front.

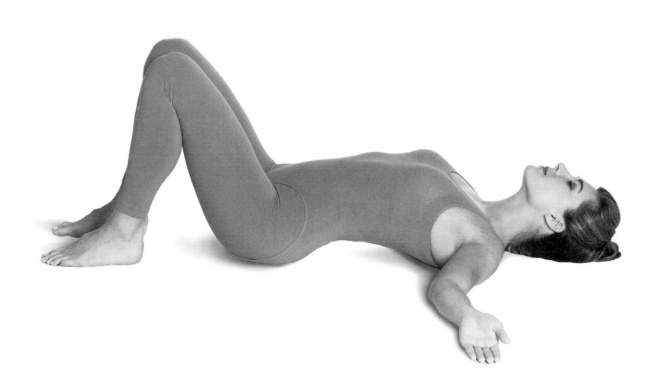

28

PARTIAL ROLL-UPS

Strengthens abdominal muscles and lower back

POSITION

Lying on your back, knees bent and feet flat on the floor, place your hands on the fronts of your thighs, pressing the small of your back flat. As you exhale, roll the upper half of your torso up off the floor, head first, only until your hands touch your knees. Press your pelvis back. Hold for a count of ten, then roll back down. Repeat, feeling the abdominals working strongly but smoothly. Do not jerk or bounce.

OBJECT

To contract the abdominals with smooth, steady pressure, in order to strengthen them so that they learn to work together with the muscles of the lower back (creating a strong natural girdle around the middle); also, to keep the pelvis pressed back during the roll up *and* down.

NOTICE

Does your neck contract as you lift up? Try to keep it loose and relaxed. Is it relatively easy to keep the small of your back against the floor? There may come a point at which you must decide whether to arch your back, to make it easier to touch your knees, or to continue pressing back and down. Don't give into the Creative Cheat of arching; keep pressing back. Press down with your feet against the floor to help keep the small of your back flat.

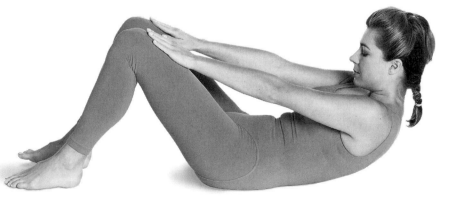

Press your pelvis back and down as you curl your upper body forward to touch your knees.

IF THIS IS IMPOSSIBLE

Make sure your pelvis is flat to the floor, as in #27. With the back of your head resting on your hands, curl up as far as you can, trying to pull forward with your shoulders and arms. Feel how the abdominal muscles must start to contract in order to do the work instead of your arms. Try to stay up a little longer each time.

IF THIS IS EASY

Reach higher and hold the position longer. Imagine a thousand-dollar bill dangling in front of your knees: as you press the small of your back down as firmly as you can, reach forward, beyond your knees, to grab the bill. You are deliberately creating a *two-way stretch,* pressing *back* toward the floor at the same time as you reach *up* with your arms. This strengthens both the abdominals and the back muscles.

Pull forward with your shoulders and arms; feel how your abdominal muscles contract as you curl up.

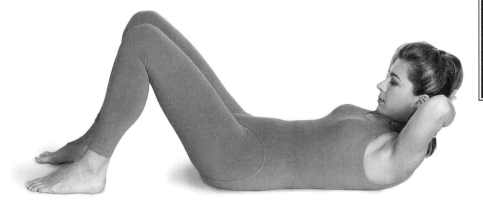

THE LOWER BACK

It's no accident that the small of the back is so often the site of pain and limitation. As we have seen, the old locked-knee way of standing shifted your weight back onto your heels, forcing your pelvis to tip forward to keep you from falling over. This retraction in the small of the back is the cause of swayback, the most common problem of misalignment.

Whenever your PAIL OF WATER is not level front to back, the muscles at the small of your back are shortened and compressed. This can be dangerous: it reduces the space between the disks in your spine, which often results in pressure on a nerve, pain and, eventually, degeneration of the disks. Lengthening the muscles in your back protects you from this, as does developing *awareness* and *flexibility* there. (The two go hand in hand: you can release a tight spot only after you become aware that it's tight and that you are responsible for holding it tight.) Now you have a choice, and you know what else you can do.

You also need to *strengthen* the muscles of the lower back, enlisting the aid of some well-developed muscles and encouraging them to work with the abdominals, so that you're held firmly upright all along your torso. This strong natural girdle of muscles around your middle, front and back will lift your torso effortlessly tall and straight. You will be able to move your spine more forward over the center of the foot, to be lifted up on the energy stream.

29

ONE-LEG ROLL-DOWN

Stretches back;
strengthens
abdominal and
lower back
muscles

POSITION

Sitting on the floor, bend one knee and grasp it with both hands, fingers laced around it. Extend the other leg out along the floor in front of you. Lean back until your arms lock straight, with pressure from the knee pulling you forward. Tilt your pelvis back (spilling water out the back of your PAIL OF WATER). Slowly roll down, placing one vertebra at a time on the floor. Lengthen your neck as you approach the floor. Roll over onto your side to return to the sitting position and repeat, until you can do the movement smoothly in slow motion on both sides.

OBJECT

To stretch the back and contract the abdominal muscles at the same time, working them together; to round the spine, using the frame of the arms and knee and the pressed-back pelvis to gain control of the entire length of the spine as it is rolled down along the floor.

NOTICE

Feel the connection between the extended leg and your back. Does the leg come up off the floor as your back reaches the point where it must round? Also, does your back want to *flatten* instead of *round* at this point? As you become more limber, the two will be independent enough that the back can round and the leg can stay down.

IF THIS IS IMPOSSIBLE

For a support to pull back against as you roll down, have someone hold your outstretched leg or place it underneath a couch or other heavy piece of furniture. *Go very slowly*, stopping at each new tilt of the vertebrae, and exhale into this place. Pull your hands forward with the bent knee to straighten your elbows. This will help stabilize you as you start to commit your pelvis to tilting backwards. Keep *extending* your spine at exactly the point where you feel weakest, and continue to press *back* with your pelvis as you roll down. This is the crux of lower-back problems:

To begin, sit very tall with a straight back.

Press your pelvis back as you begin your roll-down.

if you cannot *round out* the place that is always compressed, you will have difficulty succeeding in this movement. Conversely, when you finally discover how to "pop out" that last vertebra so that it *lengthens* when you need it, you will have successfully reprogrammed that area, going a long way toward erasing chronic back pain.

IF THIS IS EASY

Do the roll-down without any support for the outstretched leg. Then try it with your arms stretched out in front, alongside your knees, not holding on. Aim for maximum slowness, smoothness and rounding, *reaching* forward as you uncurl backwards. Maintain awareness of each vertebra separately touching the floor.

ADVANCED VERSION

One-Leg Roll-Up. From the floor, grasp one knee with both hands and roll slowly up to a sitting position. Keep the extended leg flat on the floor; place it under the couch if you need support. Notice where there may be a hitch, an interruption, in the smooth roundness of the curve of your spine. Press *back* farther into your back at that point and breathe into it. It's more difficult to roll up without a hitch than to roll down; pull against the

extended leg that is hooked under the couch (or being held down for you), and feel the transfer of weight through your thighs. If this is not enough support, go back to the One-Leg Roll-Down until the whole movement is smooth. Reverse legs. Repeat.

To make this more difficult still, let go of your knee, keeping your hands reaching out near your knees. Use *the two-way stretch* to really work the abdominals and lower back, going down and up.

Slowly roll down, holding your bent knee, touching one vertebra at a time to the floor until your back and neck are flat on the floor.

Lengthen your neck fully as you approach the floor, facing forward.

THE VANCE STANCE

Strengthens abdominal and lower back muscles

POSITION

Sit with your knees bent and your feet flat on the floor. Your arms are extended out in front of you, reaching forward. Press your pelvis back and roll down in slow motion, keeping your spine curved and continuing to reach forward with your hands. If this is easy, then roll up the same way; if not, do the One Leg Roll-Up to return to a sitting position.

OBJECT

To continue strengthening the lower back, using the abdominals as energy extends out from the hands. Using the abdominals in this way, rounding the back as you reach forward, prevents the Creative Cheat of arching the back forward, which dangerously compresses the small of the back.

NOTICE

Is there a point at which you lose control and roll back too quickly? This is the precise point where your abdominals need strengthening and your spine needs stretching.

As you roll down, continue to reach forward with your hands.

Press the small of your back flat as you roll down to the floor.

IF THIS IS IMPOSSIBLE

Hold on to your legs for support when you feel that you're losing control, then let go as you continue down. Feel how you press back as you reach forward to get past that point. Roll up, using the One-Leg Roll-Up, then roll back down with both legs bent.

IF THIS IS EASY

Make sure you're really pressing your spine back into a smooth round. Slowly and smoothly, roll your pelvis back as soon as you can when rolling down and keep it down to the last when rolling up.

ADVANCED VERSION

Roll up as well as down, maintaining the same very rounded spine. Press forward with your hands throughout.

Once you're able to roll down to the floor, roll up, maintaining a rounded back until you reach a sitting position.

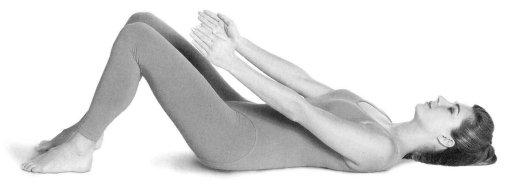

THE VANCE STANCE

Strengthens abdominal and lower back muscles

POSITION

Lying on your back, pull your knees toward your chest. Press the small of your back flat against the floor. Place your arms at your sides, flat on the floor, with your palms up and shoulders back and down. Extend your legs straight out at an angle toward the ceiling, locking your knee joints by tightening your thighs and pointing your toes.

Keep the small of your back flat against the floor. Exhale as you hold your legs straight out to a count of three. Inhale, bend your legs and bring them back in. Rest. With your back flat, repeat the movement as many times as you can do it correctly.

OBJECT

To strengthen the abdominal and lower back muscles by using the legs as a lever; to train the legs and back to work both independently and together.

NOTICE

Does your back arch up off the floor as you extend your legs? Do you get cramps in your feet or calves as you point your toes? Try to keep pressing your back down even if you must raise your legs to do so. (The narrower the angle of your legs to the floor, the stronger your abdominal muscles must be to keep your back flat on the floor. Raising your legs toward a ninety-degree angle with the floor makes less demand on the abdominals.)

Keep the small of your back flat on the floor; don't let it arch.

Release cramps by flexing the feet and legs; then resume the point.

It is essential to do this movement *exactly* as described; don't surrender to the Creative Cheat of arching your back where it is weakest when your legs are extended. Trying to support the weight of your legs with weak abdominal muscles shifts the demand to your back and could strain it. Keep the abdominals and the back muscles working together, if necessary raising your legs higher off the floor to reduce the strain.

IF THIS IS IMPOSSIBLE

If you have difficulty straightening your legs at all, and cannot even straighten them in the air (even at a ninety-degree angle to your body), lie perpendicular to a wall and place your heels up against it. Feel where you must stretch and lengthen to allow your lower back to rest down on the floor.

Then take your legs away from the wall, noticing what muscles must now engage to keep them in the air. If your problem is keeping your back flat while you extend your legs, practice the three previous movements (#28, #29 and #30) until your abdominal muscles are stronger.

IF THIS IS EASY

Make sure the back of your neck is long and that you're exhaling completely, with relaxed neck and shoulders.

ADVANCED VERSION

At each extension and exhalation, lower your legs a little. Stop at just the point where you begin to feel your back wanting to arch off the floor. This is how low your legs should go for now, and no lower. Bend your knees and bring them in, then straighten them a few times, concentrating on feeling the abdominals working; keep your neck long and strongly point your legs and toes.

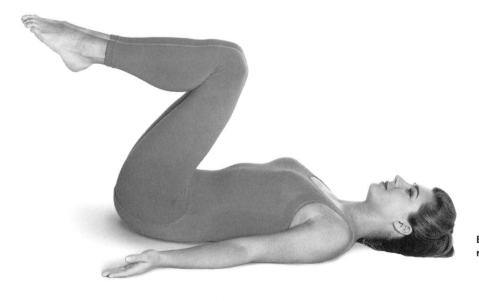

Bring your legs in toward your chest and rest between leg extensions.

32

REVERSE BRIDGE

Alternately contracts and lengthens back muscles

POSITION

Lie flat on your back, knees bent and feet flat on the floor, hip-width apart. Tuck your pelvis under, flattening the small of your back against the floor, your neck long, arms out to the sides and palms down. Gently tip your pubic bone up toward the ceiling *without lifting* any part of your back off the floor. Feel the internal angle of your groin tip up in this position, without letting your buttocks leave the floor.

Now roll the rest of your pelvis and your hips up off the floor, continuing to lengthen the small of your back as you roll higher. Maintain the angle in the crotch. Then roll your spine down along the floor from your neck first, laying down each vertebra one by one.

Repeat, continuing to lengthen your neck as you lower yourself back down.

OBJECT

Slowly, and with control, to work through each segment of the spine, contracting and stretching it in sequence from top to bottom, gaining awareness and control in an area that is often too weak for the supporting work it must do.

Tuck your pelvis under, then gently tip your pelvic bone up toward the ceiling without letting your buttocks leave the floor.

Roll your pelvis and hips off the floor, pushing up with your buttocks but keeping your torso in a straight line.

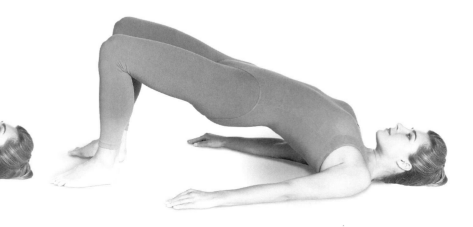

NOTICE

Do your heels tend to come up off the floor as you reach the highest point in the bridge? Press them down, directing the stretch more up into your back through your legs.

As you roll down, can you get your waist to touch the floor before your buttocks do? You must keep *lengthening* your back in order to give your waist room enough to press out, touching first. The waist is often the weakest point of the torso, where the back is the most retracted and the stomach the flabbiest.

IF THIS IS IMPOSSIBLE

Roll-Up: Begin by simply tilting your pubic bone up while your buttocks stay on the floor, then come back down flat onto the floor. Keep extending your neck out at the same time. This will lengthen your lower back, preparing you to do the whole roll, up and down. Check that your hands can just touch your heels; walk your heels in closer if you need more help in getting your hips up.

Roll-Down: Shift the weight in your hips a little forward and toward your feet as you begin to roll down. Imagine that you're peeling your spine down along the floor, while still maintaining the pressure in your legs and heels, pressing your hips up.

IF THIS IS EASY

After your roll-up, rise up on your toes, lifting your heels off the floor. Then lift your hips higher. Now, from this new height, lower your heels to the floor and roll down.

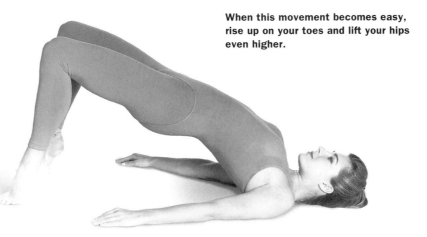

When this movement becomes easy, rise up on your toes and lift your hips even higher.

Strengthens
muscles of the
sides and upper
abdomen

POSITION

Lie on your back with your hands clasped behind your head, elbows out to the sides and shoulders down. Curl up, bringing your knees toward your chest. Point your toes and lift your head. Now touch your right elbow to your left knee, pulling your shoulder across your chest. Extend your right leg fully with the toes pointed, to just above the floor. Lock the knee. Reverse, touching your left elbow to your right knee and extending your left leg. Do not roll back down between twists; keep going, right elbow to left knee, left elbow to right knee, exhaling as fully as possible each time you touch a knee, to a count of forty.

OBJECT

To strengthen the muscles of the sides and upper abdomen as well as those of the thigh and buttocks, using the extended leg as a lever to help work the midsection.

NOTICE

Does the extended leg not want to stay straight? Or stay down low? This is a sign of weakness in this area. Is it hard to get the elbow to touch the knee? Then the stomach needs the previous work to get more strength. Do you run out of steam before you reach the count of forty? If so, reduce the number of reps at the beginning, gradually increasing until you've built up more stamina.

Keep your extended leg locked and just above the floor.

IF THIS IS IMPOSSIBLE

Hold your knee in with one hand clasped around it; support your head with the other hand. Now touch your knee with the elbow of the arm that is supporting your head. Then try to extend your leg. Switch sides.

IF THIS IS EASY

Aim higher up the arm, so that you get more contraction in the middle, and try to touch your knee with the opposite shoulder. Then switch, keeping tall in the torso as you change from side to side.

ADVANCED VERSION

Let your arms drop down at your sides and touch your knee to your shoulder without using your hands.

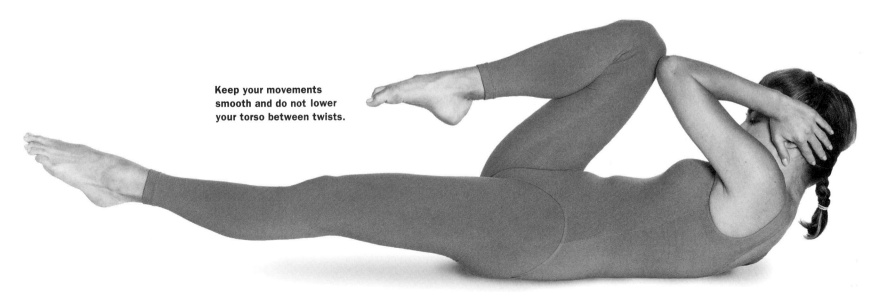

Keep your movements smooth and do not lower your torso between twists.

THE VANCE STANCE

Stretches muscles of the back and waist, releasing the neck, shoulders and arms

POSITION

Lying flat on your back, arms out to the side and palms up, bring your knees up to your chest. Drop your knees over to one side and turn your head to face in the opposite direction, keeping your shoulders flat on the floor. Return to the starting position, exhale, and repeat in the opposite direction.

OBJECT

To stretch and release the back and waist area by twisting in the midsection; to uncover hidden tightness between the hips and arms; to release in the neck and shoulders and down the arms.

NOTICE

Does the opposite shoulder lift off the floor when you drop your knees to the side? Are you unable to keep your legs together as they drop to the side, or does neither leg touch the floor at all? If so, you're tight in the hips, across the top of the chest, and in the shoulders, arms and back.

Keep your shoulders flat on the floor as you drop your knees to the side.

IF THIS IS IMPOSSIBLE

If the arm of the raised shoulder is flailing about off the floor, move your hand down until it can rest on the floor. From here, try to relax the shoulder and arm, extending outward to the outstretched hand. When you can relax at this point, sneak the forearm up the floor a little and drop into the stretch at this point. Wait, exhaling into the tightness.

If you're very tight in the hips, place one hand on the top leg and gently press it down as you continue twisting in the opposite direction. If you are really frozen, immobilized, place a cushion under your arm or between your legs until you can relax into that tightness in the hip.

IF THIS IS EASY

With your hands still on the floor, bring them closer to your head so that they're not perpendicular to your torso and legs but form an angle; keep your shoulders back and down. Make sure your legs are higher than your waistline. Roll your head farther in the direction opposite your legs, increasing the twist in your waist. Feel the stretch all the way up your spine, from tailbone to neck.

ADVANCED VERSION

When your head and shoulders can stay really flat, extend your legs out at a right angle with your torso until you can grasp your toes with your extended hand. Feel a nice stretch as you straighten your legs against the pull of your hand on your toes.

Your head and knees should always face in opposite directions.

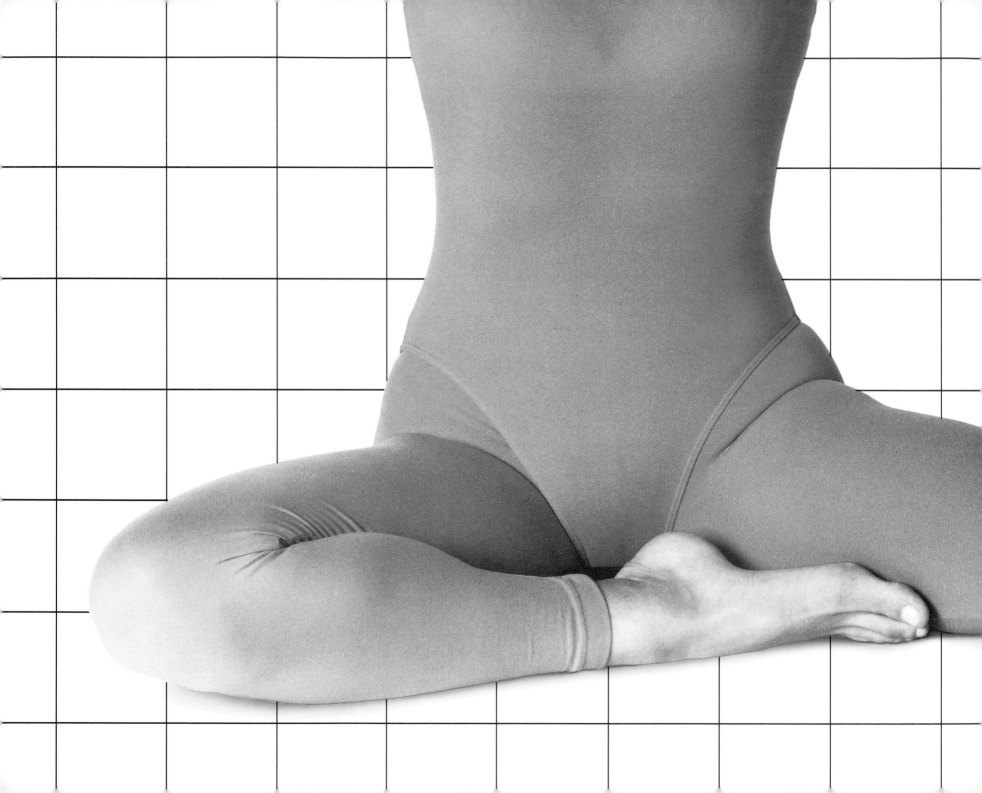

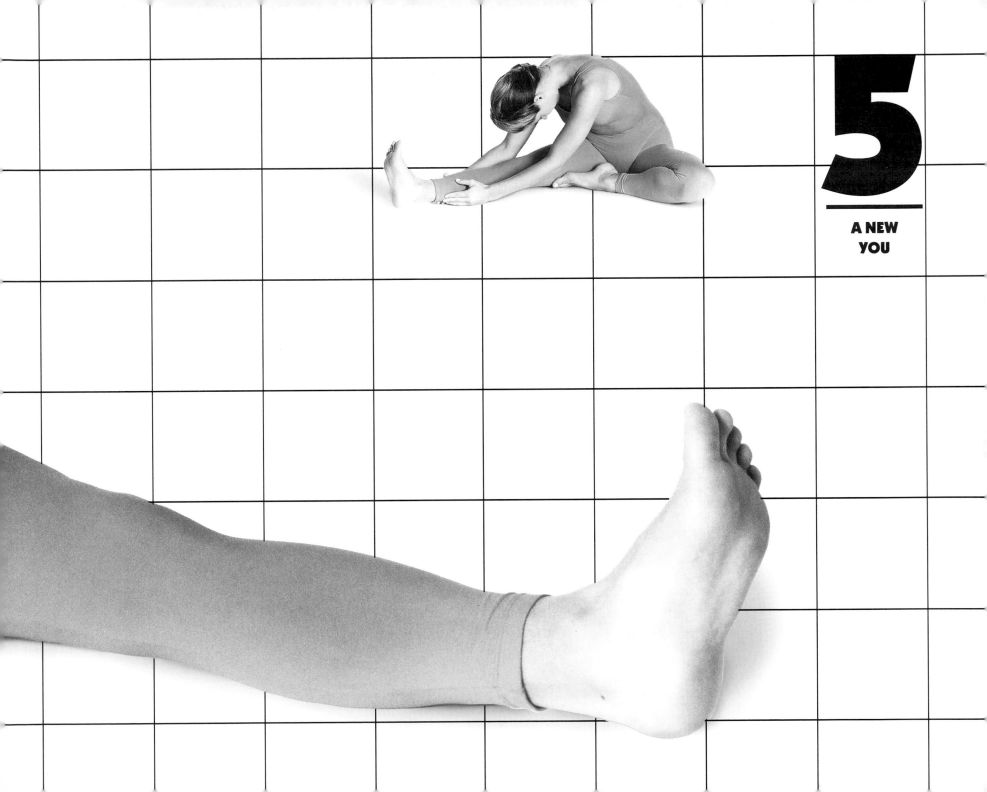

5

A NEW
YOU

CHAPTER FIVE

A NEW YOU

All your hopes and wishes, all your good intentions, won't bring about the changes you want in your body unless you actively work to make them happen. At least half my job is to help you become the kind of person who can take over the responsibility for following the program on your own, because this is how you'll achieve the kind of body you want—limber, strong, full of energy and capable of meeting every demand. And this means incorporating the Balanced Alignment of the Stance, together with the Thirty-Four Movements that facilitate it, into your everyday life as you walk, sit, stand, drive your car or engage in sports or other activities.

It is an odd paradox that the more we need the relief of stretching and releasing to restore elasticity to our muscles, the less we may feel like doing what needs to be done. In most of us, the body's feedback system seems to fail at this point. But it is this *acceptance* of stiffness and limitation that contributes most to the downhill skid so many of us enter in our forties and fifties, or even at a younger age. Happily, however, there's another side to it: the habit of stretching can become an addiction, so that the more we do, the more we feel like doing. A habit of this kind is beneficial because it involves awareness, which opposes the fixed, unthinking habit of bad use that the Vance Stance is specifically designed to help you recognize and overcome.

Getting past the barrier of initial resistance is the hardest part. After that, the habit of *wanting,* and *expecting,* to feel good takes over. Instead of downhill to decrepitude, it's clear sailing with the exuberance of new energy and new power, as well as new ease and well-being, thanks to new flexibility and balance. And you can choose to continue exploring new frontiers

ONLY YOU IN YOUR BODY

There is no one else but you inside your body. No one else knows what it's like to be inside your skin. Only you can feel where you're stiff and aching; only you can sense the connections among tensions, can track causal links between past illness or injury and present pain and limitation.

As you gradually establish the Stance as your new way of being-in-your-body, it is you who will experience the fading away of the old harmful ways of standing and moving as they are replaced by the healing "rightness" that relieves pain and eliminates the effects of the old way—even to watching bunions disappear! Once you've developed a reliable sensory awareness of what you're actually doing and how you're doing it, no one else can do as much for you as you yourself can. And only you can feel exactly where you're tight as you focus your breath in doing a movement. You inhabit your body; it's up to you to transform it.

My promise to you is that if you begin the process of transformation, a newly supple, strong and youthful body will be yours for life.

of skill in any activity—anything at all that you do with your body, from woodworking, to playing a musical instrument, to karate—with your new powers of conscious awareness and a reliable feedback system that tells you when you're off and when you're right on target. This feedback lets you know that you are now a person who is *naturally* flexible and balanced—that the "old" you, the one that seemed to be clumsy or hurting or tired most of the time, is not you anymore.

But becoming the "new" you means instilling new habits to replace the old, and this requires attention and persistence. Pain can be a great motivator; if you've suffered enough, and been debilitated enough, chances are you'll persist at anything that brings relief. If physical pain was your main reason for beginning this program, keeping pain at bay can be a strong impetus to continue. If fear of growing feeble and stiff as you get on in years was your main reason, you know now that you can have quite a lot of control in this area. You can be certain that if you exercise and move your body correctly, you will improve daily.

ADDICTION TO WELL-BEING

So let's instill this positive addiction to feeling good instead of bad. You've begun to explore the differences between the way you used to stand and move and the new way that you've been introduced to in the Stance. You have a suspicion that there may be a better way. The new "right" way is beginning by now to feel a little right, rather than strange or wrong, and you now have an idea of how to access the sensations of this new, better way.

We'll also use some simple tricks to circumvent the tendency to procrastinate—which we all have, even with regard to something that serves our own well-being. These tricks will help you get past that barrier and to the point where you've become a "stretcher," a person whose body/mind actually *craves* the sensation of stretching.

This is what we're aiming for. *We want your "appetite for stretching" to become as urgent as the appetite for eating and sleeping.* When this occurs, the issue of will power becomes irrelevant.

- Do as much of the work as possible at home. Don't wait until you've joined a gym; that time is too difficult to organize and find. One of the biggest advantages of the Vance Stance program is that it can be done entirely at home, with next to no equipment, using existing places such as a doorway or countertop.

- Get yourself a buddy, an exercise partner, and set up a support system: a phone call twice a week, or an arrangement to do the movements together, or an agreed-upon penalty if you don't each do the work—whatever it takes to get you both on the floor three times a week for fifteen minutes.

- Do the movements at the same time every day. Your unconscious mind will then be primed to take you into the exercise "mode" at that time, so that it becomes an automatic routine that you swing into—like brushing your teeth. (Alternatively, you may be a "spontaneous" exerciser, able to get into the mode, or mood, on the spur of the moment. This is hard for most people, but it does work for some of my students.)

Eventually you may be able to do the whole set of movements. For now, just do part of it—but do it *regularly.* Don't let yourself skip a session entirely just because you can't do a long, intense workout. Make a point of doing *some* movements, even if it's the Toe Crunches while you're watching TV or the Stork Stand while waiting for the water to boil.

- Spend as much time as you can on the floor. Play with your children or grand-children. You can be doing the floor exercises while you play a game of checkers, for instance.

- Sit on the floor when you watch TV and use the timing of the programs to set yourself mini-goals—a stretch during the commercial, for example, or until the next commercial break.

It's strange to me that some people think they can force themselves to exercise as a way of life. Perhaps some people can keep continually bullying themselves, but I am not such a person. Nor are my clients who work on their bodies regularly at home, by themselves, doing it by using will power. What we are doing is much more natural and much easier—we are following our desire, our appetite.

AN APPETITE FOR STRETCHING

Most of what we do that's good for us we keep on doing because nature gave us an *appetite* for it. We eat because we're hungry; any concern we may have about proper nutrition comes a long way after the sensation of hunger and the pleasure of satisfying that urge. Often we take a bath or shower just because it feels so delightful; our skin tingles, we feel refreshed, relaxed and revived. We lie down in our comfortable beds, sighing with the pleasure of stretching out between cool sheets and warm blankets, not so much because we experience biologically the need to shift into another level of brain activity (sleep, for example) as because it feels so good. We experience our needs as desires, and that's what propels us.

I propose that everyone has an innate *appetite for stretching*, along with an appetite for food or sleep, but we've learned over the years to ignore the body's cues to satisfy that appetite. (Just as we found it more expedient to choose one way of standing when we first learned to walk, our early survival required that we learn to override this appetite. But survival *now* dictates that we uncover, and use, this mechanism.) The result, as we've seen, is weak, tight or flaccid muscles. Ignoring the appetite for stretching also eventually deadens the message from the body that it *wants* to stretch. When you watch cats or dogs, they seem to be stretching most of the time they're awake. No one has to tell them that stretching is "good" for them; they experience a luxurious sense of release in the act of stretching itself, and so they do it instinctively.

Now that you've come this far, your body, mind and emotions are ready to serve you as the responsive unit it was designed to be. As we've progressed through the Vance Stance, you've probably begun to experience new feelings in new places. You are developing a new awareness of your body. Small, subtle messages that you might have ignored or perhaps not even received in the past stand a better chance of being heard now with your increased sensitivity to what's going on with your body.

And these messages include the signals from your body that it *wants* to move and stretch in this beneficial and enjoyable new way. Your feelings and sensations are now coming into sync with what your body needs and wants. The unpleasant sense of having to *force* yourself will diminish.

SEEING RESULTS

BARBARA'S STORY

Barbara, a woman in her late forties who is a fairly accomplished skater, offers a good example of the power of moderate but regular discipline. When she joined my group classes one summer, she was a pleasant-looking size twelve, a bit plump here and there, and with no muscle definition. She looked as if she could easily add five or ten pounds a year—and probably would. She was in no pain and was relatively limber, but for her frame she was too heavy and flabby.

When she returned the next summer, we all gasped in amazement: she had gone from a size twelve to a size eight! Weight control? Aerobics? Weight lifting? "No, I did Vance's movements," she told the class, "three times a week for fifteen minutes. The work I did here made me realize that if I didn't take action, I could only get fatter and fatter. And I saw enough difference in myself to convince me that change *was* possible. So I just decided to tackle it, to go ahead and do this for myself. I knew no one else could. So *I* did it, for *me*. And fifteen minutes is nothing. I just put on some Fifties music and dived in. The time flew."

A LIFELONG HABIT

To be permanently effective, the Stance and the Thirty-Four Movements that make it possible must become *a permanent part of your life*. This is both bad news and good news. Bad because it's *you* who must take the responsibility for doing them and *do* them—no getting around that.

Good for the same reason—your well-being is in your own hands, and the means to accept and succeed with this responsibility also comes from sources within yourself.

It's like that circus tumbling act in which two clowns grasp each other's ankles and roll along, each in turn pulling the other over and up. As you pull yourself, to begin with, by your intellect ("Yes, it's a good idea to start taking care of myself— I'll give it a try"), you are then pulled by the sensations in your body ("This feels good— I like it"), and the self-generated energy of the circle keeps you in motion. Round and round you're pulling/being pulled by yourself: your emotions, once you've enlisted them on the side of success (not only feeling good, but also the sense of personal control and competence), contribute their own weight. ("Wow, I'm actually becoming the kind of person who stretches and exercises—never thought I'd do it!") Once you're in the loop, momentum keeps you going.

MIND, BODY, EMOTION

Through years of working with my students, and on myself, I've learned that the most efficient way to change the body includes transformation on these three different levels: *mind, body* and *emotion.* As a tall, thin teenager with tight hamstrings and a swayback, I discovered the hard way, through trial and error, that changing my own posture meant not only changing many of the ideas I had about myself, but also confronting the emotions that surrounded those ideas. Intellect (mind) came to my aid when my sensations were still unreliable; I could tell, looking in the mirror, that what I was *doing* was wrong, even though it *felt* right. How could it be that I was standing "wrong"? What was "right"? Did anyone know how to correct this crooked, tight body? Emotions ran high as I struggled with confusion and self-disparagement. The body was the arena for all this turmoil: it was the way in, and the way out, as I began to make changes.

I discovered that the structural changes followed effortlessly once psychological blocks were uncovered and worked through, and I developed the Vance Stance to include transformation on all three levels. It's always surprising and exciting to realize how intimately the mind, the body and the emotions are connected; change in any one always accelerates and intensifies change in the other two. As a stool rests on three legs, each stabilizing the whole, so these components work together to focus our awareness.

HOW TO DO IT ON YOUR OWN

The first requirement for becoming a person who instinctively, naturally stretches, and seeks *opportunities* for stretching, is the realization that you and your body are on the same side—that you are not adversaries. When my clients first come to me, they are almost never on easy terms with their bodies. I constantly encounter a sense of conflict, as if for them it's a matter of "me" against "my body," and they must either dominate it or be dominated by it.

WHATEVER IT TAKES

At first, in order to bypass every resistance that your mind may throw in your way, you'll have to be very flexible in your approach to finding an entry point around the resistance. Know that it's normal and natural for your body not to want to change (it must have been doing *something* right to have brought you this far). Planning for the resistance will allow you to try several creative ploys. Your job is to run through your new bag of tricks until you hit on the method that works; using trial and error, you'll see which one happens to engage you long enough so that you'll persist until you feel a subtle shift.

Different things will work on different days. One day it might be bribery ("I'll let myself read that new magazine after I do the Ankle Sit for ten minutes"); the next, coercion ("No movie unless I've done three exercises"). Today's ploy may never work again—or perhaps just not until next week. The point is to keep attempting to find whatever it takes to get you to *do* something, no matter how small. Like stringing a pearl necklace, each tiny effort will add up to something great.

With this attitude, it's no wonder they dread having to work on their own bodies, on themselves, by themselves, rather than delegating the job to a masseur or chiropractor. They feel as if they're being asked to deal with an opponent they neither like nor respect. But, as we've seen, it's essential that every part of yourself—*mind, body, emotion*—work in full cooperation for your self-correction and self-improvement to work. Only then can you finish the race strong and vital. Survival is no longer enough; we expect and can now have an interesting, fun and stimulating old age. We will continue to improve, and our experience of life will be allied with an undiminished, even enhanced mastery of ourselves. We will not, and need not, permit ourselves to slide passively toward frailty and helplessness.

MOTIVATING YOURSELF

How can you set it up so you can experience an appetite for stretching in the first place, so that you can then respond to it? Here is where the tripod of mind, body and emotion comes to your aid. As with the circus tumblers, someone (or some part of you) has to start the ball rolling. That

Success lies in the united effort of mind, body and emotion.

part is the intellect, the mind. First you *recognize* and *acknowledge* that there will be hurdles to get over; thus, you allow for the most difficult part of *learning how to learn*. You are assessing the *reality* of the situation and taking conscious, intelligent steps to ensure your safe passage through the shoals of self-motivation. Alerting yourself to predictable pitfalls also reinforces the relationship of trust among the three parts of yourself.

As you establish a closer rapport with your emotional side, you may become aware of feelings of inferiority, perhaps even of stupidity and worthlessness, but you now begin to put these feelings into perspective. You begin to be able to distinguish between the "you" who is struggling to program in new pathways for yourself and the "you" who is watching and

judging and criticizing. I'll never forget what it was like watching myself beginning to learn to play polo at the age of thirty-six. I had already taken up ice hockey at thirty and karate at thirty-five, so I had an idea of what I might have to contend with in the way of self-criticism. Every day I had to keep telling myself that I was *not* merely stupid whenever I missed the ball or couldn't keep my horse in a trot as I circled around the ball. It took every bit of mature self-love I could muster to remind the child part of myself that not being able to *do* anything right at that moment was not all there was to me. Only by being aware that this old message was running rampant in me—and that it *was* an old, outmoded and senselessly hurtful message— was I able to avoid succumbing to the bad feelings I was generating in myself.

Over and over, I saw the other polo players greatly inhibit their progress in learning a new skill as they berated themselves for being what they considered "too slow" with their learning speed. My students have seen the same: it takes as long as it takes, and negativity will only hinder your progress. Bad self-talk seems to "gum up" the learning mechanism. So don't be a nagging parent to yourself; be a loving and encouraging one!

The body is both the easiest and the hardest leg of the tripod. It is the easiest in that it's the arena we think we know the best. Actually, it's simply the most apparent. It's right *there,* "real," under our noses, so to speak. Perhaps one day we will come to see how much we still have to learn about this wondrous machine. But the body is where we can most easily see and feel concrete changes, which you will bring about as you practice the Stance and the Thirty-Four Movements. When you can finally touch your hands to the floor in the Hang-Over, for example, you have actual, concrete proof of change. You have undeniably advanced!

Yet it is this very concreteness of the physical that makes it difficult to change at first. The body requires, most essentially, sheer *persistent repetition.* However disciplined your mind, you still have to *move your body* in the new paths a certain number of times in order to learn to perform any new movement easily. Just as the Black Belt in karate speaks of doing "five hundred kicks," repeating a move over and over until a certain sense memory is instilled permanently in the muscles, there is no substitute for actually doing the Thirty-Four Movements. Think how much time and how many repetitions went into forming your present habits of holding yourself in a particular way; certainly it took time for them to become *unconscious* habits. So it will take time and repetitions to undo them—though, happily, not as long or as many as went into forming them, because now you have *awareness* and *purpose* on your side.

Doing the movements precisely and with complete awareness throughout is far more important than the number of times you repeat them, and a precise awareness as you do them will bring about the changes you want far more

quickly than performing many mindless repetitions. But you *must do* them regularly!

THE JOURNEY AND THE GOAL ARE ONE

Realizing that a large part of the journey toward personal growth is the actual trip itself is of vital importance. If you don't focus too fixedly on your destination, you can enjoy each moment along the way. This takes the pressure off having to "get" somewhere. What you experience along the way becomes as interesting as where you think you're going. This is especially true in work as intrinsically pleasurable as yours. When you begin to feel the pleasure inherent in the act of stretching, you'll naturally seek to do it more and more. Like the cat and dog, you'll look for opportunities to stretch whenever you can, to feel the pleasure of the release. This is the state I am promising you,

that someday you will naturally decide to do for yourself, on your own, movements to release and strengthen your body.

The difficulty comes with all the resistance that surrounds getting to this place, but the work we have already done should have prepared you to accept that no one else can "give" it to you—and that, luckily, you can "give" it to yourself. Like self-esteem and self-love, no one acquires it from some source "out there." It has to come from within.

THE PROCESS IS THE POINT

The process of discovering your blocks and resistances will become interesting and rewarding *in itself.* True, you do have a long-range goal of self-transformation by becoming a "stretcher," but you'll also have several more immediately attainable ones along the way.

Again a critical paradox: the more directly you aim at a goal, the more difficult it is to stay in the moment and to experience the feedback of pleasure needed to continue the work long enough to reach your ultimate goal! In order to keep yourself interested and participating, there must be some sort of visible proof that you have progressed. You need small, attainable points of achievement as measurable indicators of progress. Without them, the part of you that needs all the encouragement it can get (an achieved goal) is denied the one thing that will keep you going long enough for the *appetite to stretch* to kick in.

As my students work on themselves, they continually reach what seems to be the limit of their abilities. They would always like to be more advanced than they are now. Yet you can only start to change from the point where you are now. Where you would *like* to be always seems to be in the distance; the further you expand your capacities, the farther ahead you can see and the more you can do. But it happens one step at a time, with the edge of dissatisfaction always ahead.

The more you do, the more you <u>can</u> do— there's virtually no limit!

I counsel my students to stop straining to be better than they are at any given moment and to look the other way—backwards. By looking back at where you have been, you can accurately gauge your progress and see that, without noticing it, you have actually attained some of your smaller goals. Eventually you will look back at where you are now in amazement that you ever thought of settling for so little! And then the point *from* which you look back in amazement will become the point you look back *to*—with the same amazement!

HELPING YOURSELF TO *DO* IT

So begin with small attainable goals. They will keep changing, and you may need to adjust them to suit your individual circumstances and temperament. For example, one day you might want your goal to be to "do any of the exercises on the floor, for ten minutes." Or, "I'll do any three exercises." Or, "I'll do the one I dislike the most, three times."

On a difficult day, to get yourself psyched up to do anything at all, you may have to settle for doing only the easiest ones or only your favorites (they're probably the same!). That may be all the stress you can tolerate on that particular day. Still, you've done *something,* even if it wasn't a full-speed-ahead killer workout. No matter. Brick by brick, you are laying a foundation for yourself. If you'd waited until all the conditions were optimal, you might wait forever to actually *do* something. People always want their schedules, and their motivation, and their energy level to be just right, before they can really plunge in and "do it right."

I can't tell you how often students will say, "I'm going to do an hour every single day." And then, overwhelmed by the enormity of their unrealistic goal, they end up doing nothing at all: it was too threatening, and too hard, so they shut down, unable to begin. This then makes them angry at themselves, which only sets up further resistance. Then they feel even worse and become still more resistant. Then they burden themselves still further with guilt for failing themselves—or me, or some imaginary judge.

It's worse than useless to make impossible demands on yourself; *regularity* is far more important than *intensity*. It's more valuable actually to *do* only fifteen minutes of stretching three or four times a week than it is to *think* of doing an imaginary hour a day and end up doing nothing.

Knowing that every day for a while you may face a new resistance, I've devised some ways to play with the work, to look for the access point that will do the trick for *this* day. Trust that there *is* one and that you *will* find it!

1 Notice where you are in the movements as you practice them. If you try to touch your toes, as in Movement #2 (Hands on Floor, Legs Straight), how far away from the floor are your fingers? Is it different from the last time you practiced the movement? In #24 (Sitting Forward Bend), how far away are your hands?

A NICE PLACE TO REST

FRED'S STORY

Fred and I had a good laugh one day as we worked through some of the floor movements. He had been working faithfully to open his ankles and hips in order to take the pressure off his damaged knees. The Ankle Sit had been his biggest challenge, requiring five pillows to approximate the folded-joint position. He'd had a great deal of release along the shin and foot and was progressing steadily but slowly. At sixty-five, he'd had surgery on both knees, one ankle and one Achilles tendon.

This day, we were joking back and forth as we worked. Finally he needed a rest, so he sat back on folded feet, Japanese style, to catch his breath. All of a sudden we both realized what had just happened: he had naturally assumed the position that had been his most difficult movement! This delicious irony, that he had progressed so far that now this was his comfort place, had us whooping with joy.

Has the distance changed from last time? When you cross your legs in #20 (Cross-Legged Sit), how far off the ground are your knees? In #18 (Ankle Sit), how many pillows do you need? Always look for any difference from the last time to encourage yourself with visible proof of your progress.

2 Notice which movements are the hardest for you. Which do you dislike the most? Which do you tend to forget to do? (These are probably the same.) Write them down, and make a point of focusing on these on certain days, perhaps on a high-energy day or when you only have time to do one or two movements. The rewards will be even greater than with the ones you like to do, for the tightest places are the most important to open and your improvement will accelerate. You may even derive a special enjoyment from the very movements you dreaded not so long ago, before deciding to work through your resistance to them. My clients come to love the most the ones they disliked the most: this seems to be how we experience our

Trust yourself and your ability to change. Soon enough, you'll have concrete proof of progress.

new access to areas that were formerly blocked.

3 Pick three movements at random, pledging to do just these, two times each, then stop for the day.

4 Pick an amount of time—say, ten minutes. See if you can do one movement for the entire ten minutes, or five minutes, or fifteen. Experiment, noticing how much progress you can make in a short time.

5 Alternatively, see how many movements you can do correctly, twice, in the space of ten minutes.

6 Decide in advance that you will achieve some goal for the day, *no matter what,* then enlist your creativity to help you find the access point for that day. Remember, there *is* some way for you to trick yourself to get down and

do something: it's up to you to keep experimenting until you stumble on what works for that day.

Right now, you possess all the tools you need for change. You have your *intellect,* which can jump-start your resolve until your organism becomes strong enough to do it without having to be "told" (and the appetite for stretching takes over). You have a *body* that will give you positive feedback in the form of new pleasurable feelings, strength and flexibility. And you have an *emotional side* that wants all your components to work together— that wants you to feel good *in* your body and *about* your body. It wants to give you what you say you want.

Whatever it takes, you will let yourself find it within yourself and have it because all the parts

of you, working as a unit, will be moving toward the common goal. The energy you wasted trying to find someone else to do it for you—and then not really getting it from them, not lastingly—will now be directed toward finding out for yourself how *you* really work. The sense of hopeless frustration will diminish as you come to trust your own self and your positive ability to change. You now know how to do whatever it takes to get yourself to stretch.

When it all finally comes together, and you experience the rewards of having decided to take charge of your own well-being, you'll feel another deep satisfaction: you will have completed the loop from thought to desire to action to results. Your body will have become your friend, and more important, you will have become its friend. The two of you are all you truly possess. The sooner you realize this, and accept yourself as your own partner for the long haul, the sooner you'll begin to live it to the hilt, in a body that is ready to live the fullest and richest life you can possibly imagine— for both of you.

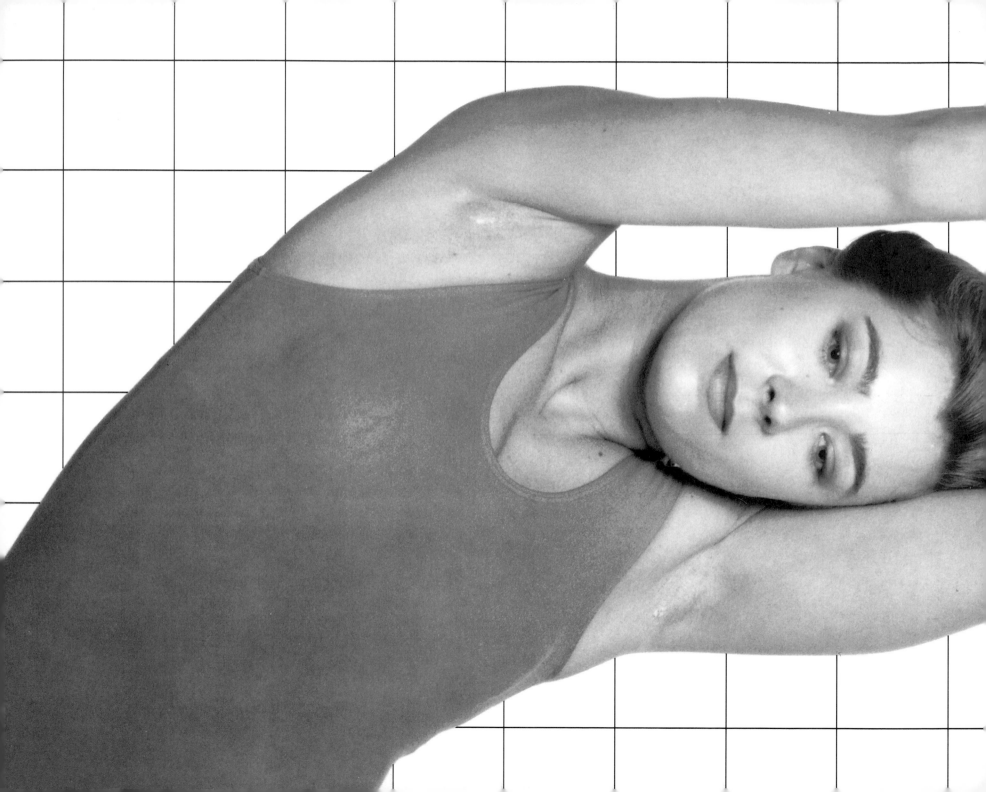

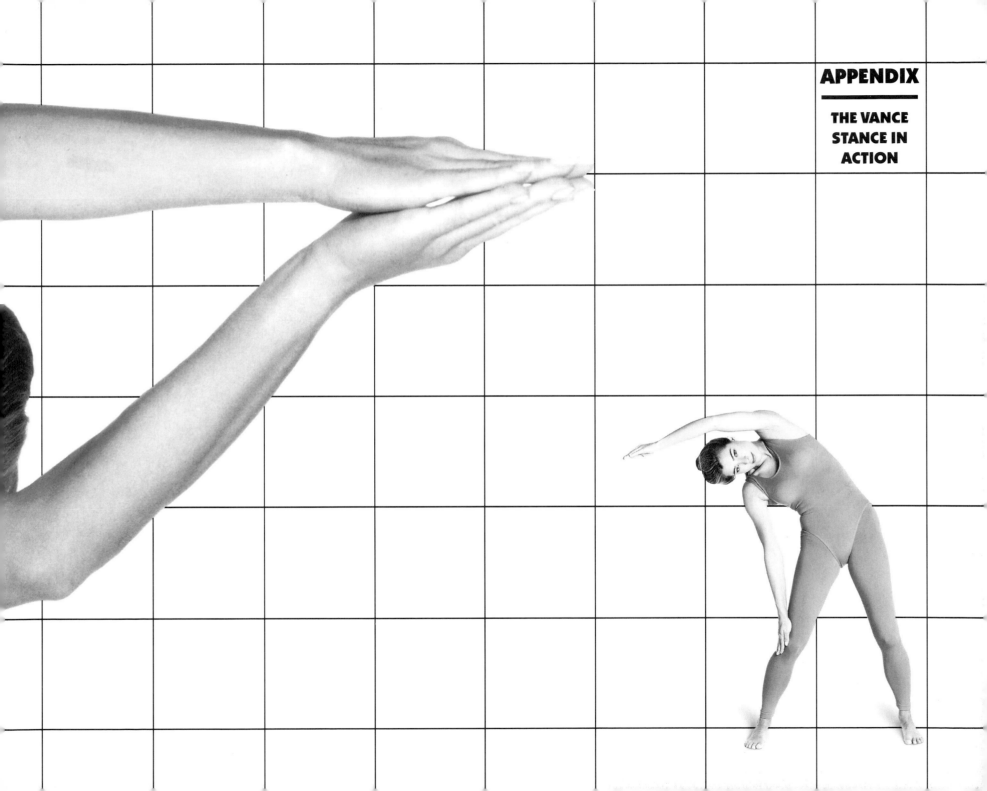

THE VANCE STANCE IN ACTION

If you have worked carefully through the Stance and gone through all of the Thirty-Four Movements at least a few times, you should now have a good understanding of how to apply the Balanced Alignment of the Stance to just about everything you do.

Using the Stance in sports and other activities is no different from using it in walking or sitting or brushing your teeth—except that the sheer excitement of sports can sometimes sweep you temporarily off course, making you lose sight of the essential relationships of Balanced Alignment that are just as vital, if not more so, to success in physical activities as they are in everything else you do.

Here are some reminders, targeted to the demands of specific activities.

● BASEBALL

Remember to keep lengthening your neck so that your head rises freely off the top of your spine. Shoulders and arms can be injured if you contract the shoulders, pulling them in, when you hit or catch the ball. To prevent this, do the following movements:

3 Doorway Stretch

14 Wrists on Railing

22 Cross-Legged Sit: Elbows Up and Out

To help keep your heels on the ground while squatting in the catcher's position, thus preventing strain in the knees:

12 Squat and Reach

● BASKETBALL

For the lift you need to jump high, open your ankles and feet with these movements:

5 Heel Drop on Stairs

9 Toe Crunch Series

18 Ankle Sit

To develop correct alignment in your legs in order to prevent strain on the lower back:

15 Stair Climb, Up and Down

● BICYCLING

Riding hunched up for long stretches tends to compress and shorten the whole body. Think, while riding, of releasing your shoulders and neck, and of lengthening your spine all the way up and out the top of your head. Even in this position, think of releasing it *into length*. Think of each of the SHIMS as being far away from the one below and the one above. Release your shoulders and let your head and neck drop forward into length whenever it's safe to do so on the road. The following movements are especially helpful:

1 The Hang-Over

3 Doorway Stretch

● BOWLING

Correct placement of the knees over the feet as you release the ball will prevent back and knee strain. To align your legs:

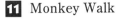 **11** Monkey Walk

16 Groucho Walk

To achieve the length needed to keep your legs aligned:

5 Heel Drop on Stairs

18 Ankle Sit

To release and lengthen your midsection:

6 Up Against the Wall

12 Squat and Reach

26 Dead Bug

● BOXING

The following movements will strengthen the abdominals:

29 One-Leg Roll-Down

31 Leg Extensions

33 Stomach Crunches

To keep light on your feet:

19 Toe Bend, Achilles Stretch

To help keep your shoulders released and down as you punch:

3 Doorway Stretch

To release your arms and back:

14 Wrists on Railing

● CANOEING

If you have difficulty sitting upright, do the following movements to stretch your back:

7 One Arm Overhead, Lean to Side

32 Reverse Bridge

To make it easier to sit in the boat with your legs folded:

24 Sitting Forward Bend

To strengthen the abdominal muscles:

33 Stomach Crunches

● DANCE

Most forms of dance encourage good alignment. However, shin splints seem to be a frequent problem of aerobic dancers, apparently caused by landing with the weight on the toes instead of on the entire foot. To help prevent this, do these movements:

9 Toe Crunch Series

Beware of the ballet dancer's walk—the "duck walk" with the toes turned out. Offstage, or outside of class, remember to keep your feet pointing straight ahead.

● FENCING

To help keep the forward leg precisely aligned over the knee:

11 Monkey Walk

12 Squat and Reach

16 Groucho Walk

To help you stand tall and easily on one leg at a time:

8 Stork Stand

To open and widen your shoulders for clear separation of your neck and arm:

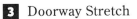 **3** Doorway Stretch

● FOOTBALL

Stretching and releasing muscles in the hips and groin will help prevent injuries. To open these areas, do the following movements:

12 Squat and Reach

21 Cross-Legged Sit: Head to Floor

26 Dead Bug

To strengthen the muscles of the thighs:

31 Leg Extensions

Be sure to stretch carefully, and cautiously, any area where you sustain an injury, especially from a blow or fall. Be careful to avoid any lasting effect from the compensations you make naturally during the healing process; be aware of what the compensations are and, as soon as the injury is healed, make a point of restoring normal Balanced Alignment.

171

● GOLF

An asymmetrical sport that stresses a one-way rotation of the body, golf needs to be compensated for by careful balancing of both sides of the body. Be especially aware of this as you practice the Stance and the Thirty-Four Movements.

To help loosen your shoulders:

14 Wrists on Railing

22 Cross-Legged Sit: Elbows Up and Out

To help lengthen your Achilles tendon, which will make your swing easier:

5 Heel Drop on Stairs

● GYMNASTICS

Beware of stressing your lower back by going swayback with exaggerated arched-back landings. To strengthen and release your lower back:

6 Up Against the Wall

27 Pelvis Flatten and Arch

● HIKING

Try these exercises on the trail.

To protect your lower back from the strain of carrying your pack and climbing hills:

1 The Hang-Over

To lengthen and strengthen your feet so that your toes can help in climbing:

5 Heel Drop on Stairs

9 Toe Crunch Series

● HOCKEY

Both ice and field

Muscle pulls in the groin are common in this sport. To stretch and strengthen muscles in this area, do these movements:

12 Squat and Reach

13 Leg on Railing

23 Head to Knee on Floor

26 Dead Bug

To release tension in your back:

1 The Hang-Over

2 Hands on Floor, Legs Straight

To release your entire spine:

24 Sitting Forward Bend

To stretch and release your feet and ankles:

5 Heel Drop on Stairs

18 Ankle Sit

● KARATE

To prevent pulling a muscle in the groin or hamstring and to open up the legs and back:

18 Ankle Sit

21 Cross-Legged Sit: Head to Floor

To release hips and lower back:

8 Stork Stand

12 Squat and Reach

26 Dead Bug

● KAYAKING

The most common problem for a beginner is lower-back strain from stretching so far in the seated position with the leg out in front.

Until the backs of your legs have stretched enough to allow the stretch up into your back:

1 The Hang-Over

2 Hands on Floor, Legs Straight

13 Leg on Railing

For the advanced paddler, dislocating a shoulder can be a risk. To lengthen and strengthen the shoulders:

3 Doorway Stretch

6 Up Against the Wall

7 One Arm Overhead, Lean to Side

22 Cross-Legged Sit: Elbows Up and Out

● POLO

Between chukkers, do the following exercises to keep your lower back flexible and supple for protection from jarring by sudden stops and shocks:

1 The Hang-Over

2 Hands on Floor, Legs Straight

To release your waist so that you can turn easily in the saddle without straining your back and to release your shoulders for fluid and powerful hits:

3 Doorway Stretch

4 Arms Behind on Railing

To stretch hamstrings and groin:

13 Leg on Railing

● RIDING

Flexibility in the ankle helps to keep you deep in the saddle. The following movements focus on flexibility in this area:

5 Heel Drop on Stairs

9 Toe Crunch Series

18 Ankle Sit

To help prevent swayback in your efforts to sit up straight:

27 Pelvis Flatten and Arch

To release tightness in the lower back:

1 The Hang-Over

To flatten your back as you release your torso upward:

6 Up Against the Wall

To release the hips and legs:

21 Cross-Legged Sit: Head to Floor

● ROCK CLIMBING

Ice and rock

Most important for flexibility and balance are open hips and flexible feet. To strengthen your feet for perching on tiny footholds:

5 Heel Drop on Stairs

9 Toe Crunch Series

12 Squat and Reach

19 Toe Bend, Achilles Stretch

21 Cross-Legged Sit: Head to Floor

26 Dead Bug

● ROWING

The following movements are helpful in training your legs to direct power smoothly from feet to hips:

15 Stair Climb, Up and Down

16 Groucho Walk

17 Up off the Floor (No Hands)

To release and strengthen your back:

30 Roll-Down, Legs Together

32 Reverse Bridge

To open your shoulders and upper back:

3 Doorway Stretch

14 Wrists on Railing

● RUNNING

It's easy to tighten in the back while running. To stretch and release this area, particularly the small of the back, do the following movements:

1 The Hang-Over

2 Hands on Floor, Legs Straight

12 Squat and Reach

13 Leg on Railing

14 Wrists on Railing

25 Knees to Chest

Knees take a lot of punishment in running if the leg alignment is not balanced. The following movements will train the knees to stay directly centered over the ankle and underneath the hip:

15 Stair Climb, Up and Down

16 Groucho Walk

17 Up off the Floor (No Hands)

● SKATING

Ice and roller skating

The more deeply you can bend your knees, the less likely you are to strain your back. Practice these movements:

15 Stair Climb, Up and Down

16 Groucho Walk

17 Up off the Floor (No Hands)

For balance:

8 Stork Stand

To release tightness in your back:

13 Leg on Railing

24 Sitting Forward Bend

To open your feet:

9 Toe Crunch Series

10 On the Ball

11 Monkey Walk

19 Toe Bend, Achilles Stretch

● SKIING, CROSS-COUNTRY

For this sport, your shoulders have to be very free of your neck. Do these movements:

3 Doorway Stretch

22 Cross-Legged Sit: Elbows Up and Out

Foot, toe and ankle articulation greatly improves your technique. To open your feet and lower legs:

9 Toe Crunch Series

10 On the Ball

11 Monkey Walk

19 Toe Bend, Achilles Stretch

To strengthen the legs:

8 Stork Stand

15 Stair Climb, Up and Down

17 Up off the Floor (No Hands)

● SKIING, DOWNHILL

The more deeply you can bend your ankles and keep your weight forward, the better. The following movements are helpful:

5 Heel Drop on Stairs

15 Stair Climb, Up and Down

17 Up off the Floor (No Hands)

18 Ankle Sit

To strengthen your midsection so you don't collapse at the waist:

6 Up Against the Wall

8 Stork Stand

To stretch your back and the backs of your legs after skiing:

13 Leg on Railing

23 Head to Knee on Floor

24 Sitting Forward Bend

32 Reverse Bridge

● SOCCER

You must be able to extend (point) your feet as well as flex at the ankles. The following movements are helpful:

5 Heel Drop on Stairs

9 Toe Crunch Series

18 Ankle Sit

To lengthen the hamstrings for high kicks:

13 Leg on Railing

23 Head to Knee on Floor

To release tension in feet and legs:

10 On the Ball

To add power for jumping:

31 Leg Extensions

● SPRINGBOARD DIVING

A strong takeoff and a tall lift with the arms and body, requires strong and open feet and legs. To strengthen and lengthen the leg muscles:

5 Heel Drop on Stairs

9 Toe Crunch Series

10 On the Ball

15 Stair Climb, Up and Down

16 Groucho Walk

17 Up off the Floor
(No Hands)

To lengthen the midsection:

6 Up Against the Wall

14 Wrists on Railing

● SWIMMING

Be sure to keep your back flat (not swayed) and your shoulders back and down. The following movements are useful in keeping the torso long and released:

3 Doorway Stretch

6 Up Against the Wall

7 One Arm Overhead, Lean to Side

14 Wrists on Railing

To develop flexibility for power in kicking:

9 Toe Crunch Series

To help release your back after you come out of the pool:

1 The Hang-Over

24 Sitting Forward Bend

● TENNIS AND RACQUETBALL

Proper placement of the knee over the foot is imperative to protect your knees.

To strengthen thigh muscles and lower legs and feet:

5 Heel Drop on Stairs

11 Monkey Walk

17 Up off the Floor
(No Hands)

To release your shoulders for more power in hitting:

3 Doorway Stretch

● VOLLEYBALL

Beach and hardcourt

Agile leaps require strong legs and flexible feet and ankles. These movements are helpful:

5 Heel Drop on Stairs

9 Toe Crunch Series

11 Monkey Walk

12 Squat and Reach

15 Stair Climb, Up and Down

16 Groucho Walk

17 Up off the Floor
(No Hands)

● WALKING

Speed and ordinary walking

If you're weak in one or both legs, you'll tend to pass the strain on to the small of your back or to your hips or knees. To practice walking at a slow-motion pace in order to learn where you may be out of balance, do the following movements:

15 Stair Climb, Up and Down

16 Groucho Walk

17 Up off the Floor
(No Hands)

For balance:

8 Stork Stand

To open your feet for takeoff and landing:

9 Toe Crunch Series

To develop awareness of the midsection muscles that support you in the upright position:

6 Up Against the Wall

27 Pelvis Flatten and Arch

To release your shoulders so that they hang freely as you walk:

3 Doorway Stretch

● WEIGHT LIFTING

Machines and free weights

Injury-free power lifting comes from impeccable alignment. Continually renew the Stance, maintaining freedom in all the muscles and especially releasing your shoulders down (keeping them dropped) for lifting and flattening your back for leg work. Keep your knees in precise alignment, especially as the weights get heavier and you increase reps.

To release your shoulders:

3 Doorway Stretch

14 Wrists on Railing

175

To strengthen your legs:

15 Stair Climb, Up and Down

16 Groucho Walk

17 Up off the Floor
(No Hands)

For your midsection:

27 Pelvic Flatten and Arch

28 Partial Roll-Ups

29 One-Leg Roll-Down

30 Roll-Down, Legs Together

● YOGA

Be careful not to hyperextend (lock) your knees or go swayback as you try to get into certain postures. Maintain Balanced Alignment in all of them (it is possible!). If you're very limber yet have a sway-back, bowlegs or knock-knees, which are common in yoga practitioners, practice the Stance extra-scrupulously to locate particular points where you may be out of alignment. The following movements are especially helpful:

6 Up Against the Wall

8 Stork Stand

13 Leg on Railing

15 Stair Climb, Up and Down

For information on Teacher Trainings, corporate seminars, speaking engagements, or private or group sessions, write to:

The Bonner System of Structural Reprograming
Vance Bonner, Ph.D.
P.O. Box 1092
Pacific Palisades, California 90272